EASY PALEO SNACKS
COOKBOOK

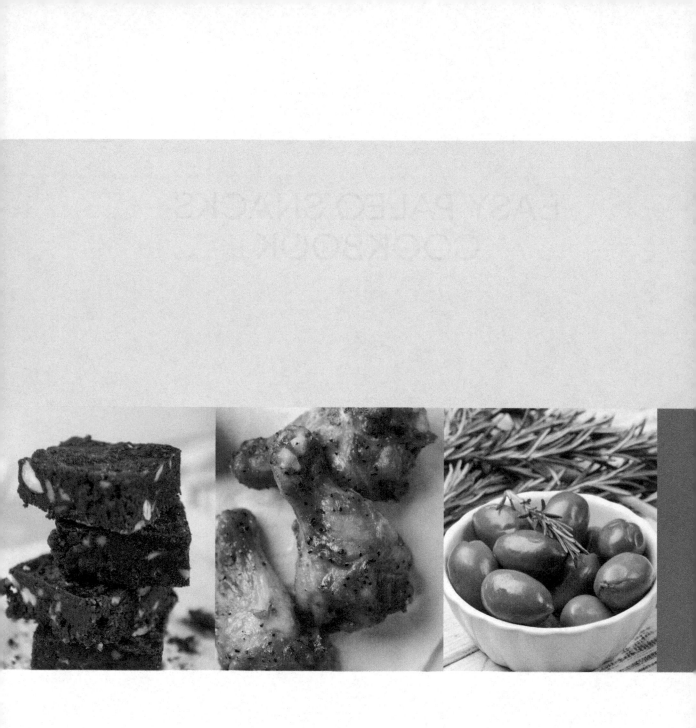

EASY PALEO SNACKS COOKBOOK

Over 125 Satisfying Recipes
for a Healthy Paleo Diet

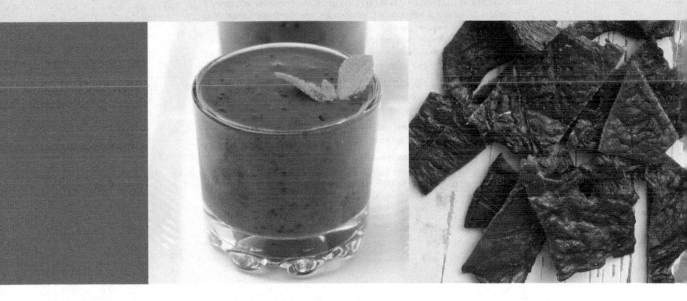

ROCKRIDGE
PRESS

CONTENTS

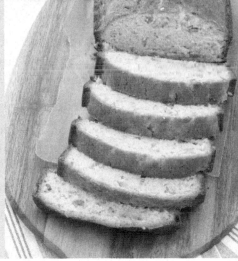

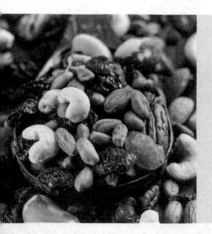

INTRODUCTION

You get it: The paleo lifestyle makes sense to you. You've done the research, read the library books, signed up for fitness and nutrition blogs, listened to a few podcasts, and even mentioned the diet to your primary care physician. You are sold on paleo. After all, how many "fad diets" date back thousands of years?

Since you've made the decision to follow this lifestyle, you've lost a few pounds, lowered your blood pressure, and even stabilized your blood sugar numbers. You have more energy and seem to sleep better at night.

Even better, you've also learned an amazing amount of new information.

You've discovered that coconuts do much more than look exotic in the grocery store. They can be turned into delicious drinks, sauces, and desserts. And you know that coconut oil can be used in cooking, not just in shampoo and tanning lotion.

You found out that garlic and onion powder aren't the only spices out there. You've cleared an entire section of your cupboard to make room for more spices, including the exotic garam masala and the spendy saffron, perhaps.

You've learned that "dark chocolate" is a vague term, but in your new lifestyle, it means at least 70 percent. You're smug when you can enjoy a piece of 90 percent and chuckle at those days when you thought 54 percent was dark!

You've learned to love vegetables you'd never even heard of before, and the produce manager knows you by your first name. You could give a 30-minute lecture on the culinary possibilities for sweet potatoes.

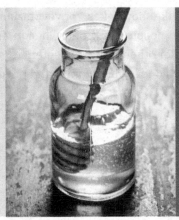

Sure, your grocery bills have gone up—buying the "real" food is definitely more expensive than the boxes and cans. However, the expenses from eating out have virtually disappeared. If you live in a large city, asking for paleo food in a restaurant may result in a few helpful suggestions. If you don't, you're probably going to have to listen to a joke about living like a caveman, and politely explain that, no, you don't usually hunt for your dinner with a spear or a large rock.

So there's only one problem: You've got meals covered, but what about snacks? You know, snacks—the food you want between your nutritious and tasty meals. The treats your kids want when they come home from school or bring a friend over. The nibbles you crave late at night when the house is quiet. The platters you want to serve when the gang comes over to watch the game.

Snacks. The "fourth meal."

On the paleo diet, it can seem impossible to find snacks to replace old favorites, but it doesn't have to be that way. This cookbook is here to rescue you from those weak moments when you hear potato chips or brownies calling your name. It has every kind of snack you could want—sweet and salty, small and large—and all quick, healthy, easy, and delicious! Each chapter starts with an "extremely easy" recipe, one that usually requires little to no cooking or any special ingredients. Nutritional breakdowns are provided so you can keep track of the calories, carbs, fat, protein, sodium, and sugar in each dish.

A note about ingredients: Just like snowflakes—or vegetarians—no two paleo dieters are exactly alike. Some people allow dairy, bacon, fermented foods (vinegar, sauerkraut), or honey or other natural sweeteners; some don't. This cookbook attempts to keep each one of you in mind and presents a variety of recipes from which to choose.

These snacks are your "missing link" in the paleo diet. Enjoy!

QUICK SUBSTITUTES AND ONLINE RETAILERS

Some of the paleo snacks in this book call for unusual or out-of-the-way ingredients. Adding just a few of these ingredients to your pantry can expand your repertoire and help you stick to the paleo diet, but there is no need to purchase all of these ingredients.

Almost every unusual ingredient has a substitute that may be more familiar. Before preparing a recipe with an unfamiliar ingredient, check the following chart and see if there is a quick substitute.

Most of these ingredients are available at natural foods co-op stores or larger natural retailers such as Whole Foods, but you can also purchase them online through specialty retailers.

 All the ingredients listed in this book with * have a quick substitute or an online retailer listed in this chart. ➤

INGREDIENT	QUICK SUBSTITUTE	ONLINE RETAILER
Agave nectar/ agave syrup	Maple syrup or honey in a 1:1 ratio	www.naturesagave.com
Almond meal/ almond flour	Other nut meal/flours such as hazelnut meal	www.nuts.com
Arrowroot	Cornstarch or potato starch	www.penzeys.com
Cake spice	Combine cinnamon, cloves, nutmeg, and allspice to equal amount of cake spice called for	www.thespicehouse.com
Coconut aminos	Bragg's amino acids, soy sauce	www.vitaminshoppe.com
Coconut flour/ coconut meal	Almond flour	www.hodgsonmillstore.com
Dried buckwheat	Quinoa	www.localharvest.org
Dried chervil	Dried parsley	www.thespicehouse.com
Flaxseed	Hemp seeds, sesame seeds or wheat germ	www.hodgsonmillstore.com
French vanilla liquid stevia/ stevia powder/ liquid stevia	Agave syrup, maple syrup	www.vitaminshoppe.com
Ghee	Butter or oil	www.ancientorganics.com
Hemp seeds/ hemp hearts	Flaxseed, sesame seeds, or wheat germ	www.manitobaharvest.com
Pink salmon roe	Bottarga, tobiko, caviar	www.houseofcaviarandfinefoods.com
Psyllium husks	Oat bran, rolled oats, wheat bran	www.vitaminshoppe.com
Seaweed — dulse and nori	Other crumbled sea vegetable such as wakame, or try salt, chopped bacon, or chopped beef jerky	www.seaveg.com
Vanilla bean paste	Vanilla extract	www.williams-sonoma.com

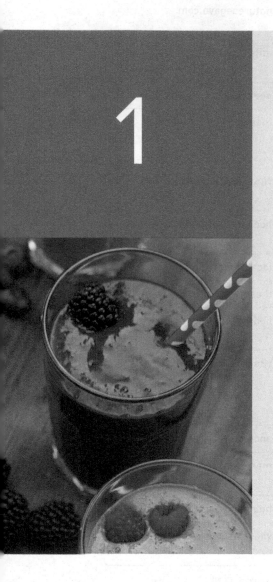

1

SMOOTH SIPPING

Sometimes being able to drink a meal is exactly what we need. Maybe we're in a hurry, maybe we don't feel like preparing a complete meal, or maybe we're just out of clean silverware. In this case, smoothies, often referred to as shakes, can be the perfect choice. They are fast and simple—you'll see that the directions are almost identical for each recipe—and easy to tailor to your preferences.

Most of these recipes are for one or two people because making smoothies for more takes mega-size blenders that most of us don't have. Just plan to make and repeat for more servings—or be generous and share yours!

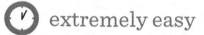 extremely easy

COCONUT DREAM

MAKES 2 SERVINGS   *Prep time: 5 minutes* • *Cook time: None*

This is the easiest, fastest, most basic smoothie for when time and supplies are running low. Make sure your coconut milk is stirred and not solid when added.

2 bananas
4 ounces coconut water
3 ounces light coconut milk
Handful of ice

1. Place all ingredients in a blender.

2. Blend until smooth.

PER SERVING Calories 210   Total carbohydrates 41g   Fat 5g
Protein 2.3g   Sodium 96mg   Sugar 26g

DOUBLE-A SHAKE

Prep time: 5 minutes • *Cook time: None*

This smoothie features exotic ingredients like ground fennel and star anise, giving it a uniquely delicious flavor that stands out from the rest. The two A's—almond milk and almonds—bring it all together.

1 cup ice
1 cup almond milk or coconut milk
1 cup plain yogurt
¼ cup slivered almonds
1 teaspoon ground cinnamon
1 teaspoon ground fennel
½ teaspoon ground star anise
Mint leaf

1. Place the ice, almond milk, yogurt, almonds, cinnamon, fennel, and star anise in a blender.

2. Blend until smooth. Serve with a mint leaf on top for garnish.

PER SERVING Calories 159   Total carbohydrates 9.8g   Fat 10.8g
Protein 7.3g   Sodium 61.1mg   Sugar 6.2g

DOUBLE-B SHAKE

MAKES 1 TO 2 SERVINGS   *Prep time: 5 minutes • Cook time: None*

Berries and bananas double the pleasure of this smoothie. The berries must be frozen to get the right texture. You can buy fresh ones in season and freeze them, or simply purchase frozen berries and enjoy this shake year-round.

1 cup frozen black raspberries
½ cup frozen blueberries
1 banana
½ cup unsweetened coconut milk
1 cup crushed ice
Few frozen berries for garnish

1. Place the frozen raspberries, frozen blueberries, banana, coconut milk, and ice in a blender.

2. Blend until smooth. Place a couple of frozen berries on the top for a garnish.

PER SERVING   Calories 217   Total carbohydrates 27.7g   Fat 12.7g
Protein 2.8g   Sodium 11.5mg   Sugar 13.6g

PROTEIN POWER

MAKES 1 SERVING   *Prep time: 5 minutes* • *Cook time: None*

This quick and simple smoothie gives you a nice punch of protein to start the day, thanks to the egg whites (don't worry—you won't taste them). Use any kind of berries you like.

1 cup frozen berries of choice
⅓ cup unsweetened coconut, shredded
½ cup almond milk
2 egg whites

1. Place the frozen berries in a blender and pulse with a bit of hot water to break up and soften them.

2. Add the coconut, almond milk, and egg whites.

3. Blend until smooth.

PER SERVING Calories 472   Total carbohydrates 28.2g   Fat 37.7g
Protein 10.8g   Sodium 133mg   Sugar 171g

DESSERT
IN A GLASS

PROTEIN

MAKES 1 SERVING   *Prep time: 5 minutes • Cook time: None*

When you're craving something sweet and a little decadent, this shake can do the trick—without guilt! The almond butter and chocolate make a perfect pair. Try not to drool on the blender lid!

3 tablespoons almond butter
¼ cup coconut milk
2 teaspoons cocoa powder
1 cup ice
3 tablespoons water

1. Place all ingredients in a blender.

2. Blend until smooth.

PER SERVING Calories 472   Total carbohydrates 28.2g   Fat 37.7g
Protein 10.8g   Sodium 133mg   Sugar 17.1g

GINGER TREAT

MAKES 1 SERVING   *Prep time: 5 minutes • Cook time: None*

Here's a smoothie that combines some unusual flavors, creating a fresh drink to kick off your day. Ginger has many health benefits, and it's lovely with pear.

1 cup pear juice, unsweetened

3 peaches, chopped with pits removed

2 tablespoons low-fat plain yogurt

1 banana, sliced

1 teaspoon finely grated fresh ginger

1. Place all ingredients in a blender.

2. Blend until smooth.

PER SERVING Calories 472   Total carbohydrates 21g   Fat 1g
Protein 2g   Sodium 13mg   Sugar 20g

FRUIT SLUSH

MAKES 2 SERVINGS   *Prep time: 5 minutes* • *Cook time: None*

Longing for one of those slushes full of artificial colors and sugar? Do your body a favor and try this one instead. It's all natural and totally refreshing. Cranberry and apple give it a tangy-sweet taste.

1½ cups frozen mixed berries
1 cup apple juice, chilled
⅓ cup cranberry juice
Handful fresh berries for garnish

1. Place berries and juices in a blender.

2. Blend until smooth. Pour into glasses and top with fresh berries.

PER SERVING   Calories 110   Total carbohydrates 23g   Fat 0g
Protein 1g   Sodium 11.75mg   Sugar 23 g

FIT WITH FIBER

MAKES 2 SERVINGS   *Prep time: 5 minutes • Cook time: None*

This smoothie tastes good, plus the psyllium husks provide your body with a healthy helping of fiber. A great way to help you and your family feel better and stay fit. Whip it up, grab it, and go!

2½ cups papaya, peeled and chopped
1 banana, sliced
½ cup plain yogurt
1 tablespoon psyllium husks*
1 cup orange juice

1. Place all ingredients in a blender.

2. Blend until smooth. Serve in chilled glasses.

PER SERVING Calories 239   Total carbohydrates 40g   Fat 3g
Protein 6g   Sodium 61.1mg   Sugar 40g

*See page 9 for quick ingredient substitutes and online retailer information

MANGO MADNESS

MAKES 2 SERVINGS   *Prep time: 5 minutes* • *Cook time: None*

Mangos are often overlooked in the produce section because people aren't sure how to eat them. Give this shake a try and chances are you'll never pass up the chance to taste this tropical fruit again. If your kids haven't tried mango yet, this makes a wonderful introduction.

1 ripe mango, peeled and chopped into chunks
1½ cups almond milk, unsweetened
½ cup low-fat yogurt
2 tablespoons almond meal*
1 tablespoon honey
Handful of ice
Honey for drizzling

1. Place mango, almond milk, yogurt, almond meal, 1 tablespoon honey, and ice in a blender.

2. Blend until smooth. Top with a drizzle of honey.

PER SERVING Calories 265   Total carbohydrates 35g   Fat 3g
Protein 15g   Sodium 0mg   Sugar 9g

---

*See page 9 for quick ingredient substitutes and online retailer information

GREEN GOODNESS

MAKES 1 TO 2 SERVINGS   *Prep time: 20 minutes* • *Cook time: None*

Not all smoothies are sweet and fruity. Try this one for a savory treat bursting with nutrition. With kale, lettuce, apple, cucumber, and more, it's a whole garden in a glass!

1 cup water

1 cup coconut water

5 celery stalks, chopped

1 large head romaine lettuce

1 large bunch kale

1 apple, cored and chopped

1 banana, chopped

½ cup chopped cucumber

½ cup cilantro

½ cup parsley

Juice of 1 lemon

4 pecans, chopped

Dash of cayenne, cinnamon, and/or
    turmeric (optional)

1. Pour the water and coconut water into a blender. Add the celery and romaine lettuce, and purée on low.

2. Add the kale and increase the blender speed. Process until well blended.

3. Add the rest of the ingredients and blend until creamy. You may add a little extra water if you'd like the smoothie to be thinner.

PER SERVING Calories 155   Total carbohydrates 32g   Fat 0g
Protein 5g   Sodium 0mg   Sugar 15g

SMOOTHIE WITH A KICK

GREEN

MAKES 1 SERVING *Prep time: 10 minutes* • *Cook time: None*

If you enjoy smoothies that are more like meals than milkshakes, give this one a whirl. Go easy on the hot sauce!

½ chopped tomato

¼ cup chopped cucumber

½ avocado

⅓ cup frozen spinach/small handful raw spinach

1 teaspoon hot sauce

½ teaspoon lemon juice

½ cup ice

1. Place all ingredients in a blender.

2. Blend until smooth. Taste to see if you want more hot sauce or lemon juice, and add accordingly.

PER SERVING Calories 148   Total carbohydrates 13.2g   Fat 10.9g
Protein 3.1g   Sodium 0mg   Sugar 0g

BEST OF BOTH WORLDS

MAKES 1 SERVING   *Prep time: 5 minutes* • *Cook time: None*

Not sure if you want something sweet or savory? With an antioxidant-rich blend of kale and blueberries, this smoothie offers a little of both. You'll get a wallop of protein, too, thanks to the whey.

½ cup frozen blueberries

¼ cup coconut water

1 stalk kale, chopped and stem removed

1 scoop whey protein powder

1. Place all ingredients in a blender.

2. Blend until smooth.

PER SERVING   Calories 166   Total carbohydrates 22.8g   Fat 1.8g
Protein 19.9g   Sodium 0mg   Sugar 7g

UBER-GREEN SMOOTHIE

MAKES 1 SERVING   *Prep time: 5 minutes • Cook time: None*

Here's a smoothie that is thick and creamy—thanks to frozen ingredients—and includes a slightly unconventional ingredient for the adventurous cook. Why not take a chance and shake things up?

1 cup unsweetened almond milk
2 cups spinach
½ avocado, frozen
½ banana, frozen
2 tablespoons hemp seeds/hearts*
Handful of ice

1. Place all ingredients in a blender.

2. Blend until smooth.

PER SERVING   Calories 357   Total carbohydrates 29.2 g   Fat 24.2g
Protein 10.4g   Sodium 235mg   Sugar 8.1g

* See page 9 for quick ingredient substitutes and online retailer information

GREEN CHOCOLATE SMOOTHIE

MAKES 1 SERVING   *Prep time: 5 minutes* • *Cook time: None*

Chocolate and spinach? Sounds crazy, but it tastes much better than you think! In fact, this may become your favorite way to get greens into your kids—or your spouse.

1 cup unsweetened almond milk

2 cups spinach

1 cup raspberries

2 tablespoons ground flaxseed*

2 tablespoons shredded coconut

1 tablespoon cocoa powder

Handful of ice

1. Place all ingredients in a blender.

2. Blend until smooth.

PER SERVING Calories 240   Total carbohydrates 26.9g   Fat 14.3g
Protein 8.1g   Sodium 235mg   Sugar 8.1g

*See page 9 for quick ingredient substitutes and online retailer information

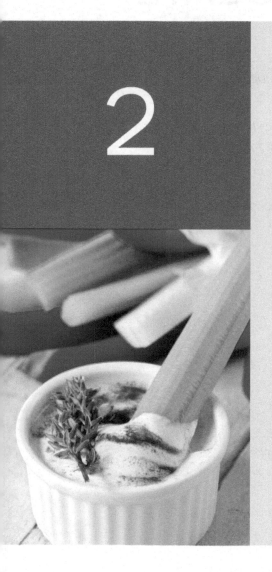

2

CHIPS AND DIPS

You may not be able to fathom how chips could be made out of vegetables like taro root, parsnips, and squash—but perhaps people once thought making chips out of potatoes sounded pretty odd. Vegetable chips are becoming more popular and can be found in many natural foods stores, as well as chain grocery stores, but be sure to check the ingredient lists for those hidden additives that so many companies slip in. You can play it safe—and have more fun—by making your own chips. This chapter gives you a variety of terrific ideas.

As for dips, most recipes out there rely heavily on sour cream, cream cheese, and mayonnaise. This chapter includes one such dip; the other three recipes use tasty alternative ingredients.

OLÉ VEGGIES!

Everyone loves to dip and crunch. One of the easiest ways to do this is with freshly cut veggies and some paleo salsa. Many store-bought brands are paleo friendly, so check their ingredient lists. (The biggest culprits will be added corn or sugar.)

Here are some good choices of vegetables:

Baby carrots

Celery stalks

Broccoli florets

Cauliflower florets

Red, green, yellow, and orange pepper slices

Jicama slices

Mushrooms

Raw sweet potato slices

Veggie chips are another great possibility for dipping into paleo salsa; try those made from parsnips, turnips, beets, and sweet potatoes.

TARO TIME

MAKES 2 SERVINGS   *Prep time: 10 minutes* • *Cook time: 30 minutes*

Taro root is one of those vegetables you have to search for carefully when you go to the store, but once you find it, you'll be glad you did. It's a cousin of the potato—kind of odd-looking, but delicious as prepared in this recipe. Serve with a sandwich or alone as a tasty snack.

1 large taro root, peeled and sliced into quarter-inch circles
1 tablespoon olive oil
½ teaspoon salt

1. Preheat the oven to 450°F.

2. Place the sliced taro in a 1- to 2-inch-deep dish. Brush the slices with the oil and sprinkle with the salt.

3. Bake until the tops of the chips are crisp, about 15 minutes.

4. Remove from the oven, flip the chips over, and put back into the oven for another 15 minutes until the other side is crisp.

PER SERVING Calories 64   Total carbohydrates 1g   Fat 6.8g
Protein 0.4g   Sodium 582mg   Sugar 0g

MAPLE SNIP CHIPS

Who would have ever thought to make parsnips into chips? This recipe does just that! A light glaze of maple syrup makes it a heavenly snack.

1 pound parsnips, peeled and cut into chip-size pieces
¼ cup coconut oil, melted
3 tablespoons maple syrup

1. Preheat the oven to 400°F.

2. Place the parsnips in an ovenproof dish, and cover with the oil and maple syrup. Stir to ensure even coating.

3. Bake for 15 minutes.

4. Remove from the oven, flip each slice over, and cook for another 15 minutes until both sides are browned. Remove and let cool for a few minutes before serving.

PER SERVING Calories 186   Total carbohydrates 109g   Fat 59g
Protein 1g   Sodium 49mg   Sugar 98g

NUTTY CHIPS

MAKES 4 SERVINGS   *Prep time: 20 minutes • Cook time: 1½ hours*

Okay—it's a trick name because there are no nuts in this dish, but it is made from butternut squash. When you add cinnamon, nutmeg, and other warm spices, it transforms into a comforting snack.

1 medium butternut squash
2 tablespoons coconut oil or ghee*, melted
½ teaspoon cinnamon
Pinch of nutmeg, ginger, cloves, and allspice (enough to make about ½ teaspoon)
Pinch of salt

1. Preheat the oven to 250°F.

2. Peel the squash and slice it very thinly, no more than ⅛ inch thick. (If you have a mandoline, that works best.)

3. Place the sliced squash in a large bowl. In a separate small bowl, mix the oil and spices together, and then pour over the squash. Stir gently until each piece is evenly coated. Arrange the slices right next to each other on a baking tray lined with parchment paper.

4. Bake for about 1½ hours or until crispy; baking time could be less, or as much as 2 hours, depending on your preference and the thickness of the chips. Keep a close eye. When brown and crispy, remove the chips and allow them to cool.

PER SERVING Calories 104   Total carbohydrates 12.4g   Fat 6.9g
Protein 1g   Sodium 16mg   Sugar 8g

*See page 9 for quick ingredient substitutes and online retailer information

CHIPS FROM THE SEA

MAKES 2 SERVINGS   *Prep time: Less than 5 minutes   •   Cook time: 5 minutes*

Need a little extra boost to your thyroid? Try this unusual chip recipe. Seaweed is a rich source of iodine and selenium, both of which are needed for thyroid hormone production. Of course, this crunchy snack from the sea is one that everyone can enjoy.

1 tablespoon sesame oil
1 cup dulse seaweed*
Sesame seeds and/or salt

1. In a large skillet, heat the oil over medium heat. Add the seaweed and heat for 1 to 2 minutes. It will turn golden brown and shrink a bit.

2. Turn the seaweed over so it heats for another minute or so, but do not let it turn black.

3. Remove the seaweed and drain on paper towels. Sprinkle some sesame seeds and/or salt over them and serve!

PER SERVING Calories 78   Total carbohydrates 12.4g   Fat 7g
Protein 1.2g   Sodium 355mg   Sugar 0.2g

* See page 9 for quick ingredient substitutes and online retailer information

TROPICHIPS

MAKES 2 SERVINGS · *Prep time: 10 minutes* · *Cook time: 15 minutes*

A new twist on the concept of chips! This fun recipe gives you a chance to use plantains—those banana-like fruits you've seen in the produce section.

1 green plantain, peeled

1 yucca root, peeled

1 sweet potato, peeled

4 tablespoons olive oil

½ teaspoon salt

1. Preheat the oven to 350°F.

2. Slice the vegetables extremely thin, ⅛ inch or less. (If you have a mandoline, that works best.) Brush both sides of the slices with the oil and place them on a baking sheet. Cover the slices with another baking sheet.

3. Bake for 15 minutes until golden brown and crispy. Season with the salt and serve.

PER SERVING Calories 405   Total carbohydrates 42.4g   Fat 24.5g
Protein 2.2g   Sodium 600mg   Sugar 0.2g

ZUKE CHIPPERS

MAKES 2 SERVINGS   *Prep time: 10 minutes*   •   *Cook time: 2 hours*

Another vegetable-turned-chip, the zucchini is incredibly versatile. It's also nutrient-dense with magnesium, fiber, and folate.

1 large zucchini, thinly sliced into rounds
2 tablespoons olive oil
1 teaspoon salt

1. Preheat the oven to 225°F.

2. Line two large baking sheets with parchment paper.

3. Place the zucchini slices in a single layer on paper towels, cover with more paper towels, and press to soak up as much liquid as possible. Line up the zucchini on the baking sheets, placing them close but not overlapping. Brush them with the oil and sprinkle with the salt.

4. Bake the chips until browned and crisp, about 2 hours. Let them cool before serving.

PER SERVING Calories 145   Total carbohydrates 5.4g   Fat 13.8g
Protein 2g   Sodium 976mg   Sugar 0g

SWEET AND SPICY CHIPS

MAKES 6 SERVINGS   *Prep time: 15 minutes • Cook time: 15 minutes*

If you like your sweet and salty mixed, this is a fun recipe that hits both cravings at once. The maple syrup contrasts nicely with the cayenne pepper.

2 tablespoons olive oil

2 tablespoons maple syrup

¼ teaspoon cayenne pepper

3 large sweet potatoes, peeled and sliced

Salt and pepper

1. Preheat the oven to 450°F.

2. Line a baking sheet with aluminum foil.

3. In a small bowl, combine the oil, syrup, and cayenne pepper. Brush half of the mixture onto the sweet potato slices, and season with salt and pepper.

4. Bake for 8 minutes. Remove from the oven, turn the slices over, brush them with the remaining mixture, and then return them to the oven.

5. Bake until tender and the edges are crispy, about 7 minutes.

PER SERVING Calories 253   Total carbohydrates 50.2g   Fat 4.6g
Protein 3.6g   Sodium 190mg   Sugar 9g

VERY VEGGIE DIP

MAKES 8 SERVINGS   *Prep time: 10 minutes* • *Cook time: None*

This is a terrific dip that works well with all types of veggies, as well as with chips. Scoop it up generously and enjoy the spicy kick.

1 cup olive-oil mayonnaise

1 teaspoon curry powder

1 teaspoon crushed garlic

1 tablespoon tarragon vinegar

1 teaspoon grated onion

1 teaspoon prepared horseradish

1. In a medium bowl, combine the mayonnaise, curry powder, garlic, vinegar, onion, and horseradish.

2. Mix them together until well blended. Serve, or chill overnight for a stronger flavor.

PER SERVING   Calories 199   Total carbohydrates 1.2g   Fat 21.9g
Protein 0.3g   Sodium 158mg   Sugar 2g

GAME DIP

MAKES 8 SERVINGS   *Prep time: 15 minutes* • *Cook time: None*

Combine olives with chiles, onions, and tomatoes, and what have you got? An accompaniment that's perfect for any chips you make, or for veggies. Prepare to double the recipe, though—your friends will eat it up as fast you make it.

2 Roma/plum tomatoes, chopped

One 4-ounce can of black olives, chopped

One 4-ounce can of green chiles, chopped

3 green onions, chopped

3 tablespoons olive oil

1½ tablespoons red wine vinegar

1 teaspoon garlic salt

1. In a large bowl, mix all ingredients.

2. Serve with chips or vegetables.

PER SERVING   Calories 70   Total carbohydrates 2.9g   Fat 6.6g
Protein 0.5g   Sodium 515mg   Sugar 0g

SALSA SENSATION

MAKES 4 SERVINGS   *Prep time: 20 minutes • Cook time: None*

Who doesn't like salsa? It's one of the most popular dips and can easily be made completely paleo. This recipe includes jalapeño, but you can add a chopped habanero pepper to really turn up the heat.

6 Roma tomatoes, chopped
½ red onion, chopped
Juice of 1 lime
½ bunch cilantro, chopped
1 jalapeño pepper, chopped
1 habanero pepper, chopped (optional—these are very spicy!)
1 garlic clove, chopped
Black pepper

1. Place the tomatoes, red onion, lime juice, cilantro, jalapeño, habanero (if using), and garlic in a food processor. Season with black pepper.

2. Blend until you get the chunky or smooth texture you prefer.

PER SERVING Calories 30   Total carbohydrates 6.7g   Fat 0.3g
Protein 1.3g   Sodium 9mg   Sugar 0g

ROASTED REDS

MAKES 6 SERVINGS   *Prep time: 10 minutes • Cook time: 20 minutes*

Red peppers are good; roasted red peppers are amazing, with their sweet and smoky flavor. Try this dip and you'll be convinced. Using jarred peppers saves time and helps you get this snack on the table quickly.

2 cups walnuts, shelled and soaked for an hour to soften

½ teaspoon ground cumin

½ teaspoon salt

One 12-ounce jar roasted red peppers, drained

1 tablespoon minced garlic

2 tablespoons olive oil

2 teaspoons lemon juice

1. Place the walnuts, cumin, and salt in a food processor. Blend until finely ground to the consistency of a thick paste.

2. Add the red peppers, garlic, oil, and lemon juice, and blend until smooth.

PER SERVING   Calories 308   Total carbohydrates 8.2g   Fat 30.1g
Protein 6.5g   Sodium 971.4mg   Sugar 1.0g

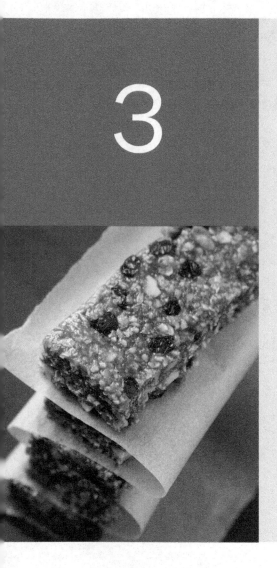

3

GRAB A BAR

Protein bars, energy bars, granola bars … whatever you call them, they're great snacks for people of all ages. And when you make them yourself, you can be sure that they're healthy. Full of fiber and protein, they're easily portable and incredibly durable. Put them in a lunch box, backpack, briefcase, or purse and you have a nutritious snack right at your fingertips.

A few of these recipes use protein powder—which some paleo fans love and some don't. Protein powder varies a great deal, so if you're going to use it, make sure you use a high-quality product made from eggs and meat (although whey protein is acceptable if you include dairy in your diet).

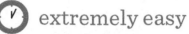

"BIRDSEED" SQUARES

MAKES 20 SERVINGS   *Prep time: 5 minutes • Cook time: 10 minutes*

At first glance, these bars may look like something that belongs in your bird feeder, but actually they're delicious treats meant for people. The birds will envy you!

⅔ cup sesame seeds
⅓ cup sunflower seeds
⅓ cup honey
⅓ cup almond butter
¼ cup flaxseed*

1. In a dry, heavy skillet over medium heat, toast the sesame seeds and sunflower seeds until they are light brown.

2. In a saucepan over low heat, heat the honey and almond butter. When warm, stir in the toasted seeds, and then add the flaxseed.

3. Line an 11-by-17-inch dish with plastic wrap and press the mixture into it.

4. Allow it to cool completely, about 2 hours. Cut into squares and serve.

PER SERVING Calories 80   Total carbohydrates 7.2g   Fat 5.4g
Protein 2.3g   Sodium 21mg   Sugar 4.65g

See page 9 for quick ingredient substitutes and online retailer information

PALEO PROTEIN BARS

MAKES 20 SERVINGS *Prep time: 15 minutes • Cook time: 1 hour 10 minutes*

Perfect for a quick energy and nutrition pick-me-up, these paleo bars are full of healthy nuts and fruit. Yes, there are many ingredients in this recipe, but the preparation is easy—and you'll find that the taste is well worth it.

2 cups walnuts	¾ cup almond flour*
1 cup pecans	¾ cup coconut flour*
2 cups almonds	¼ cup maple syrup
1 cup pumpkin seeds	3 tablespoons coconut oil
1 cup dried cranberries	2 teaspoons vanilla extract
½ cup pitted dates	1½ teaspoons cinnamon
½ cup raisins	1½ teaspoons molasses

1. Preheat the oven to 225°F.

2. On a baking sheet, spread the walnuts and pecans in a single layer. Bake until the nuts are roasted, about 30 minutes. Remove from the oven and turn the heat up to 250°F.

3. Grease a 9-by-13-inch baking pan.

4. Place the roasted walnuts and pecans, plus the almonds, in a food processor, and pulse until the mixture has a coarse meal texture. Add all of the other ingredients and pulse until well combined. Press the mixture into the greased pan.

5. Bake until golden brown, about 40 minutes. Cut into 20 bars.

PER SERVING Calories 356 Total carbohydrates 25.4g Fat 25.2g
Protein 12.5g Sodium 53mg Sugar 18.7g

* See page 9 for quick ingredient substitutes and online retailer information

A COCONUT DATE

MAKES 4 SERVINGS   *Prep time: 10 minutes* • *Cook time: None*

Cashews—yes or no? The answer depends on which paleo follower you ask. This recipe puts cashews to use in a great way, so if they're on your definite "yes" list, whip up these bars and enjoy.

½ cup slivered almonds
½ cup coconut flakes
10 pitted dates
¼ cup cashews
1 teaspoon coconut oil

1. In a food processor, blend the almonds and coconut. Add the dates and pulse until all ingredients are combined.

2. Add the cashews and oil, and pulse again until the mixture is thick and begins sticking together.

3. Transfer the mixture to a sheet of wax paper and form into an even square. Chill in the refrigerator for at least 30 minutes. Cut into 4 small squares and serve.

PER SERVING   Calories 249   Total carbohydrates 22.9g   Fat 17.3g
Protein 4.5g   Sodium 61mg   Sugar 17.6g

NATURE'S CANDY BARS

MAKES 6 SERVINGS   *Prep time: 10 minutes* • *Cook time: None*

These bars are great for energy—but they taste so good, they seem more like dessert. There's even a bit of cocoa powder here for chocolate lovers. Be sure to give the bars time to chill.

1 cup chopped dates
¾ cup almond butter
½ cup flaked coconut
3 tablespoons unsweetened cocoa powder
Pinch of salt

1. Place all ingredients in a food processor and blend until smooth and very sticky, about 4 minutes.

2. Line a loaf pan with wax paper and press the mixture into it.

3. Chill in the refrigerator for 30 minutes. Remove from the pan and slice into 6 bars to serve.

PER SERVING Calories 308   Total carbohydrates 33.2g   Fat 18.5g
Protein 9.5g   Sodium 231mg   Sugar 27.4g

BB BALLS

MAKES 12 SERVINGS   *Prep time: 15 minutes • Cook time: None*

When your sweet tooth is calling and you need a little boost, try these delicious BB Balls. Though they're not technically "bars," they can simply be flattened to become squares or can be rolled as directed here. Fresh blueberries are best in this recipe, but frozen, thawed berries can be used instead.

4 dates, pitted
1 cup walnuts
½ cup macadamia nuts
2 tablespoons coconut oil
½ cup blueberries
½ cup unsweetened shredded coconut or sesame seeds, divided

1. In a food processor, blend the dates until they form a paste.

2. Add all of the nuts and blend again, 30 to 40 seconds. With the processor blades still moving, slowly add the oil until blended.

3. Transfer the batter to a medium bowl, and add the blueberries and ¼ cup coconut. Form the batter into balls.

4. Place the remaining ¼ cup coconut in a small bowl. Roll the balls in the coconut until coated. Have a couple right now or put them all in the refrigerator for later.

PER SERVING Calories 340   Total carbohydrates 22g   Fat 29g
Protein 5g   Sodium 55mg   Sugar 18g

CINN–NUT CRACKERS

MAKES 12 SERVINGS   *Prep time: 30 minutes* • *Cook time: 15 minutes*

Okay, these aren't actually crackers, but close enough. Great alone or with dip, or alongside your cup of coffee, they're full of antioxidants and protein, thanks to the walnuts.

2 cups walnuts

1 teaspoon baking soda

¼ teaspoon salt

3 teaspoons ground cinnamon

2 tablespoons melted butter

1 tablespoon honey

1 tablespoon water

1. Preheat the oven to 375°F.

2. In a food processor, pulse the first four ingredients until finely ground, about 45 seconds.

3. In a separate bowl, mix the melted butter, honey, and water until a smooth paste is formed.

4. Line a baking sheet with parchment paper, smear the batter onto it, and shape it into a rectangle about 11 by 8 inches.

5. Bake for 12 to 15 minutes until browned. Let it cool completely and then cut into 12 pieces.

PER SERVING Calories 309   Total carbohydrates 9g   Fat 30g
Protein 6g   Sodium 49 mg   Sugar 1.1g

NO-BAKE BARS

MAKES 6 SERVINGS   *Prep time: 5 minutes* • *Cook time: None*

Perfect for an on-the-go snack or a treat at recess, these protein-rich bars don't even require any baking time—simply mix the ingredients and press into a pan. Easy breezy.

½ cup flaxseed meal*

2 tablespoons coconut flour*

2 tablespoons sesame seeds

10 tablespoons whey protein powder

3 tablespoons unsweetened cocoa powder

⅛ teaspoon stevia powder*

⅓ cup almond butter

2 tablespoons coconut oil

1 teaspoon vanilla extract

½ cup water

1. In a large bowl, combine all of the dry ingredients.

2. In a medium bowl, mix the almond butter and oil. Add to the dry ingredients and mix well. (Try a spoon—but your hands will probably work best.) Add the vanilla and water, and mix thoroughly.

3. Grease a 9-by-9-inch pan and press the dough into it. Chill in the refrigerator for about 2 hours. Cut into 6 pieces.

PER SERVING   Calories 197   Total carbohydrates 6.2g   Fat 18.0g
Protein 5.2g   Sodium 344mg   Sugar 0.8g

See page 9 for quick ingredient substitutes and online retailer information

CHERRY CHUNK BARS

MAKES 9 SERVINGS   *Prep time: 10 minutes* • *Cook time: None*

Dried cherries give these bars a sweet-tart tang while delivering a boost of antioxidants. Shredded coconut and two kinds of nuts provide a satisfying texture and crunch. Grab a few to take to work.

1 cup raw almonds

½ cup raw walnuts

1 cup dates, pitted

¾ cup whey protein powder

¼ cup unsweetened cocoa powder

½ teaspoon salt

¼ cup dried cherries

¼ cup shredded coconut

1. Place all of the nuts in a food processor, and process until they are ground into meal.

2. Add the dates and process, and then add the protein powder, cocoa powder, and salt. Transfer the mixture to a large bowl.

3. Mix in the dried cherries by hand. Press the dough into the cups of a muffin tin. Sprinkle shredded coconut on top and chill in the refrigerator overnight.

PER SERVING Calories 190   Total carbohydrates 18.6g   Fat 12.4g
Protein 4.8g   Sodium 181.7mg   Sugar 13.4g

GREEN BARS

MAKES 8 SERVINGS   *Prep time: 10 minutes* • *Cook time: 30 minutes*

Vegetables are so much more adaptable than we give them credit for, and these zucchini bars prove it. As an after-school snack, they're a great way to sneak a few more veggies into your kids.

¾ cup butter, softened

½ cup honey

¼ cup maple syrup

2 eggs

1 teaspoon vanilla extract

1¾ cups coconut flour*
   or almond flour*

½ teaspoon salt

1½ teaspoons baking powder

2 cups grated zucchini

¾ cup shredded unsweetened coconut

¾ cup raisins (plumped in hot water
   and drained)

1. Preheat the oven to 325°F.

2. In a large bowl, cream together the butter, honey, syrup, and eggs, and then add the vanilla.

3. In another large bowl, sift together the dry ingredients and then add them to the creamed mixture. Stir in the zucchini, coconut, and raisins, and then spread the mixture into a greased jelly roll pan.

4. Bake for 30 to 40 minutes until lightly browned and a toothpick inserted in the center comes out clean.

5. Allow to cool and cut into 8 bars for serving.

PER SERVING Calories 170   Total carbohydrates 18.5g   Fat 4.5g
Protein 2.3g   Sodium 133.5mg   Sugar 9.6g

See page 9 for quick ingredient substitutes and online retailer information

NUTTIN' HONEY BARS

MAKES 24 SERVINGS   *Prep time: 25 minutes • Cook time: 30 minutes*

These honey-walnut bars are pretty sweet and rich—especially with the icing, so use it sparingly—but you'll enjoy every bite. They're sure to be a hit with your family.

For the bars:

½ cup butter, softened

¼ cup coconut oil

1 cup honey

1 teaspoon baking powder

¼ teaspoon salt

3 eggs

1 teaspoon vanilla extract

1½ cups coconut flour*

1 cup shredded unsweetened coconut

1 cup walnuts, chopped

For the icing:

¼ teaspoon vanilla extract

1 tablespoon coconut milk

1 teaspoon stevia*

Chopped walnuts

To make the bars:

1. Preheat the oven to 350°F.

2. In a large mixing bowl, beat the butter and oil with a mixer on medium to high speed for 30 seconds. Add the honey, baking powder, and salt, and beat until thoroughly mixed. Add the eggs and vanilla, and beat until thoroughly mixed. Stir in the coconut flour, shredded coconut, and walnuts.

3. Spread the batter into a 13-by-9-by-2-inch pan and bake for 30 minutes. While the bars are cooling, make the icing. ➤

*See page 9 for quick ingredient substitutes and online retailer information

To make the icing:

1. Mix the vanilla, milk, and stevia until the icing is thin enough to drizzle over the bars.

2. Drizzle the icing over the top of the cooled bars, sprinkle with chopped walnuts, and cut into 24 pieces.

PER SERVING   Calories 205   Total carbohydrates 25.2g   Fat 11.2g
Protein 2.5g   Sodium 86.6mg   Sugar 8.3g

BAR NONE

Is it a breakfast bar? Is it a dessert? It could be both! Try it and see for yourself. You'll love the blend of seeds, almonds, and raisins. Agave nectar adds a touch of sweetness.

1¼ cups blanched almond flour*

¼ teaspoon salt

¼ teaspoon baking soda

¼ cup grapeseed oil

¼ cup agave nectar*

1 teaspoon vanilla extract

½ cup shredded coconut

½ cup pumpkin seeds

½ cup sunflower seeds

¼ cup slivered almonds

¼ cup raisins

1. Preheat the oven to 350°F.

2. In a small mixing bowl, combine the almond flour, salt, and baking soda.

3. In a larger bowl, combine the grapeseed oil, agave nectar, and vanilla. Stir the dry ingredients into the wet mixture. Add the coconut, seeds, almonds, and raisins, and stir to combine.

4. Grease an 8-by-8-inch baking dish with grapeseed oil. Press the dough into it and flatten it out evenly. (Put a little oil on your hands first and it will stick less to you and stay more in the dish.)

5. Bake for 20 minutes. Allow to cool, and then slice into 12 bars.

PER SERVING   Calories 146.6   Total carbohydrates 6.5g   Fat 12.6g
Protein 3.5g   Sodium 86.1mg   Sugar 3.8g

---

* *See page 9 for quick ingredient substitutes and online retailer information*

PECAN PARADISE

MAKES 12 SERVINGS   *Prep time: 10 minutes   •   Cook time: 50 minutes*

Craving a piece of pecan pie? Try this and enjoy the flavor without any of the guilt.

1¾ cups almond flour*

3 eggs

1 tablespoon coconut oil

½ teaspoon arrowroot*

¼ teaspoon salt

8 ounces dates, pitted

¼ cup maple syrup

½ teaspoon vanilla

1 cup pecans, chopped

1. Preheat the oven to 350°F.

2. In a food processor, combine almond flour, 1 egg, coconut oil, arrowroot, and salt and process until it becomes a stiff dough.

3. Using your hands, press the dough into an 8-by-8-inch pan. Bake for 15 to 18 minutes.

4. While the crust is baking, blend the dates in a food processor on high for 1 minute. Add the remaining 2 eggs, syrup, and vanilla, and process on high until smooth.

5. Pour the mixture into the baked crust and sprinkle the pecans over the top. Gently push the nuts into the topping.

6. Return the pan to the oven and bake for 30 to 35 minutes. Allow to cool before cutting into 12 bars.

PER SERVING   Calories 161.9   Total carbohydrates 20g   Fat 8.9g
Protein 2.8g   Sodium 67.3mg   Sugar 16.3g

See page 9 for quick ingredient substitutes and online retailer information

BUCKWHEAT BARS

MAKES 32 SERVINGS *Prep time: 10 minutes • Cook time: 40 minutes*

Wait! What? Buckwheat? How can that be in a paleo book? Simply put, buckwheat is the fruit seed of an Asian dock plant. Is it technically paleo? The verdict is still out on that, but if you're straddling a few lines, having relatives over, or making the transition, why not start here?

1 cup dried apple

½ cup dried apricot

2 cups raisins, divided

½ cup dried buckwheat*

1 cup water

2 cups unsweetened apple juice

2 teaspoons cinnamon

1 teaspoon vanilla extract

¼ cup butter

1½ cups coconut flour or almond flour*

2 cups sliced almonds

2 cups shredded coconut

1 egg

1 teaspoon baking powder

½ cup applesauce

¾ cup honey

1. Preheat the oven to 350°F.

2. Place the dried apple and apricot, 1 cup raisins, buckwheat, water, juice, cinnamon, and vanilla in a large pot. Bring the contents to a boil and stir until the mixture is creamy and thick. Add the butter and stir until it is thoroughly mixed. Remove the pot from the burner.

3. Add the remaining 1 cup raisins, flour, almonds, coconut, egg, baking powder, applesauce, and honey. Stir until it is completely mixed and has the consistency of cookie dough. If the batter is too thick, add an egg. If it's too thin, add some flour.

4. Divide the batter between two greased 9-by-13-inch pans. Bake for 25 minutes, until golden brown. Allow to cool and cut into 32 squares.

PER SERVING Calories 148.8   Total carbohydrates 24g   Fat 6g
Protein 2g   Sodium 42.5mg   Sugar 19.8g

*See page 9 for quick ingredient substitutes and online retailer information

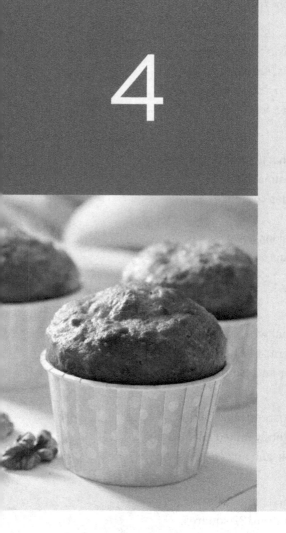

4

JUST FOR KIDS

Without a doubt, one of the best ways to help your kids jump onto the "paleo bandwagon" is to get them involved in the process. Have them help you find recipes and try them out. Take them to the store with you and have them pick out the ripest fruit or the best bargain. Cook and bake together in the kitchen. Let them experiment now and then—an involved child is almost always a cooperative child. These recipes will get you started.

A safety note: Whether you do the chopping and slicing or allow your kids to do it is a judgment call that you, the parent, have to make. The same goes for taking pots and pans on and off the stove top or into and out of the oven. If your child is young and has little experience in the kitchen, plan to make each of these recipes together. Having fun is essential—but so is staying safe.

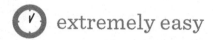

COCOFRUIT

MAKES 3 TO 4 SERVINGS   *Prep time: 15 minutes* • *Cook time: None*

Keeping a child's attention for long, complex recipes can sometimes be challenging. If you are just starting to cook with your child, or if you want to give your little one a recipe to make alone, this recipe is a good starting point.

The nutritional breakdown for this dish is almost impossible, since you decide, from one time to the next, what to put in it. With fruit and coconut milk, however, there are no worries or surprises. It's all good for you.

Have your child decide what type of fruit and nuts to include in the recipe, or use whatever fruit is in season or on special at the store. Suggestions include apples, oranges, bananas, grapes, cherries, berries, and melons. This recipe is a great way to experiment with unusual or exotic fruit, too.

Fruit of your choice, chopped

8 ounces coconut milk

½ cup shredded unsweetened
   coconut

½ cup nuts of your choice, chopped
   (walnuts, pistachios, almonds,
   macadamia nuts, pecans)

Dash of spices of your choice
   (cinnamon, allspice, nutmeg)

1. As you chop the fruit and nuts into bite-size pieces, have your child measure out the coconut milk and stir it to a smooth consistency.

2. Your child can then place the chopped fruit in a large bowl, add the chopped nuts and coconut milk, and stir it up.

3. Have your child sprinkle the shredded coconut and spices on top, and serve.

PANCAKE SURPRISE

MAKES 2 SERVINGS   *Prep time: 5 minutes • Cook time: 5 minutes*

When you read these ingredients, you may be skeptical: How in the world can they turn into a pancake? It's true, they do—and kids will have a great time making a pile of them. Grab the maple syrup!

1 banana, mashed
1 egg
1 teaspoon arrowroot powder*
Maple syrup, almond butter, coconut flakes, or nuts for topping

1. Place all ingredients in a blender, and blend until well mixed.

2. Heat a large nonstick skillet over medium heat, and ladle half of the batter into it. Cook for 2 to 3 minutes until bubbles appear.

3. Flip and brown the other side; then repeat with the other half of the batter.

4. Put on a plate and top with maple syrup, almond butter, coconut flakes, or nuts.

PER SERVING Calories 93   Total carbohydrates 14.9g   Fat 2.7g
Protein 3.8g   Sodium 36mg   Sugar 13.4g

See page 9 for quick ingredient substitutes and online retailer information

NUTRI-MUFFIN

MAKES 16 SERVINGS • *Prep time: 10 minutes* • *Cook time: 25 minutes*

These muffins taste good enough to be dessert, but they pack an amazingly nutritional punch. Carrots, dates, and bananas add up to a flavorful treat.

2 cups almond meal or almond flour*	1 cup dates, pitted
2 teaspoons baking soda	3 eggs
1 teaspoon salt	1 teaspoon apple cider vinegar
1 tablespoon ground cinnamon	¼ cup coconut oil
3 ripe bananas	1½ cups carrots, shredded

1. Preheat the oven to 350°F.

2. In a large bowl, combine all of the dry ingredients.

3. In a food processor, mix the bananas, dates, eggs, vinegar, and oil. Combine the wet mixture into the dry ingredients; then fold in the carrots.

4. Spoon the batter into greased muffin tins and bake for 25 minutes.

PER SERVING   Calories 144.7   Total carbohydrates 14.3g   Fat 3.3g
Protein 3.8g   Sodium 288.7mg   Sugar 8.5g

* See page 9 for quick ingredient substitutes and online retailer information

MIRACLE MUFFIN

MAKES 1 SERVING   *Prep time: 5 minutes • Cook time: 1 minute*

This bakes so fast that kids are often as fascinated by the process as they are by the taste of the muffin. It's a simple recipe, but so delicious.

¼ cup almond flour*
2 tablespoons flaxseed meal*
1 large egg
½ teaspoon coconut oil
½ teaspoon ground cinnamon
¼ teaspoon baking powder
Pinch of salt

1. Lightly grease two microwave-safe baking dishes , such as custard cups or ramekins.

2. In a large bowl, combine the almond flour, flaxseed meal, egg, oil, cinnamon, baking powder, and salt. Divide the mixture between the two greased baking dishes.

3. Heat the dishes in the microwave on high for 30 seconds, let rest for 5 seconds, and then heat again for 30 seconds. Remove the dishes and flip upside down onto plates to cool.

PER SERVING Calories 285   Total carbohydrates 13.8g   Fat 18.4g
Protein 20.1g   Sodium 586mg   Sugar 0g

*See page 9 for quick ingredient substitutes and online retailer information

NUTS 'N' SPICES

MAKES 4 SERVINGS *Prep time: 5 minutes • Cook time: 10 minutes*

Mixed nuts are a great snack with lots of protein, but most of the store-bought varieties are covered in too much salt or sugar. Here's a way to make your own and send it along in lunches or give for after-school snacks. You can eat these immediately after making them or store them in an airtight container for a week or so.

1 cup hazelnuts
1 cup walnuts
1 tablespoon butter
¼ teaspoon salt
¼ teaspoon ground cinnamon
¼ teaspoon ground nutmeg
Zest of 1 orange

1. Preheat the oven to 375°F.

2. Mix the nuts together in a bowl and place them on a baking sheet. Bake for 10 minutes.

3. Meanwhile, in a skillet over medium heat, melt the butter, and as it begins to brown, add the salt, cinnamon, nutmeg, and orange zest.

4. Add the toasted nuts to the saucepan and mix until thoroughly coated.

PER SERVING Calories 268   Total carbohydrates 6g   Fat 27g
Protein 6g   Sodium 140g   Sugar 0g

COCOSQUASH

MAKES 4 SERVINGS   *Prep time: 15 minutes*   •   *Cook time: 10 minutes*

If you've been struggling to get your child to appreciate squash, try this recipe. It might just change some minds and become a family favorite.

½ butternut squash

1½ cups coconut milk

¼ teaspoon ground cinnamon

¼ cup pecans

Nuts of your choice, butter, maple syrup, or coconut flakes for garnish

1. Cut the squash in half (always have an adult do this, as squash is very tough and takes muscle to cut). Scoop out the seeds and pulp, and then peel the outside. Cut the squash into chunks, place in a microwave-safe bowl, and heat on high for 6 minutes, or until soft.

2. Place the squash in a food processor, and blend until smooth. Add the coconut milk and cinnamon and blend thoroughly.

3. Pour into bowls and garnish with extra nuts and a bit of butter, a drizzle of maple syrup, or some coconut flakes.

PER SERVING   Calories 292   Total carbohydrates 15g   Fat 27g
Protein 4g   Sodium 0g   Sugar 3g

OFF TO BRUSSELS

MAKES 6 TO 8 SERVINGS   *Prep time: 10 minutes* • *Cook time: 11 minutes*

When it comes to vegetables, Brussels sprouts have a lousy reputation. Cooked the wrong way, they can taste like soggy old cabbages. But when they are prepared well, they're delicious. Have your kids give this dish a try and see if they improve their attitude about this vegetable.

1 cup water

Two 10-ounce packages frozen Brussels sprouts

¼ cup butter

8 ounces walnuts

3 tablespoons honey

¼ teaspoon ground allspice

¼ teaspoon ground nutmeg

¼ teaspoon salt

1. In a saucepan, bring the water to a boil and add the Brussels sprouts. Return to a boil, reduce the heat, and simmer, covered, for 5 to 7 minutes.

2. Once the sprouts are tender, drain them.

3. Place the butter, walnuts, honey, and spices in a microwave-safe bowl. Cover and cook on high for 3 to 4 minutes until the butter is melted. Stir to combine.

4. Pour over the Brussels sprouts and serve.

PER SERVING Calories 326   Total carbohydrates 16.6g   Fat 28.1g
Protein 8.1g   Sodium 140mg   Sugar 11.3g

PEAS-FULL SOUP

MAKES 5 SERVINGS   *Prep time: 20 minutes • Cook time: 15 minutes*

Thick, rich, and nutritious! You'll need a pressure cooker for this one, but your kids are sure to have fun helping you prepare and eat it. The bacon adds wonderful flavor to this pea soup.

2 garlic cloves, minced

1 onion, chopped

2 celery stalks, chopped

3 tablespoons olive oil

1¾ cups dried split peas

Two 14.5-ounce cans chicken broth

1 bay leaf

2 strips of bacon, chopped

2 carrots, chopped

2 teaspoons dried chervil*

Salt and pepper

1. Using a pressure cooker over medium heat, sauté the garlic, onion, and celery in oil for 5 minutes. Add the peas, broth, bay leaf, and bacon.

2. Cook under pressure for 10 to 12 minutes.

3. Once the peas are soft, stir in the carrots and chervil, and simmer for 15 minutes. Season with salt and pepper. If the soup is too thick, feel free to add a little water.

PER SERVING   Calories 509   Total carbohydrates 70.5g   Fat 15.2g
Protein 24.9g   Sodium 663mg   Sugar 12.3g

* See page 9 for quick ingredient substitutes and online retailer information

KALE KAPER

Kale is one of the most nutritious foods on the planet. It's high in iron, protein, and fiber, as well as vitamins A, C, K, and B$_6$. Yet, if you serve it to people—especially kids—chances are they'll leave it on their plates in the hope it's just a large garnish. This recipe is one way to try kale that just might convert a few people in your household.

1 bunch kale, stems removed and leaves chopped

1 teaspoon salt

2 apples, diced

¼ cup olive oil

⅓ cup dried cranberries

⅓ cup toasted, unsalted sunflower seeds

2 tablespoons raw apple cider vinegar

⅓ cup crumbled Gorgonzola cheese

1. In a large bowl, rub or massage the kale gently with salt until the leaves begin to wilt.

2. Gently stir in the apples, oil, cranberries, sunflower seeds, and vinegar until all ingredients are evenly mixed.

3. Gently fold in the cheese, and serve.

PER SERVING   Calories 142   Total carbohydrates 12.7g   Fat 9.5g
Protein 3.6g   Sodium 308mg   Sugar 10.5g

FRUITY FREEZE

MAKES 6 SERVINGS   *Prep time: 10 minutes • Cook time: None*

This is quick, is easy, and tastes especially good on a hot summer afternoon—or when you're missing one in the middle of winter. Make sure to use ripe bananas for the best flavor.

2 ripe bananas, mashed
¼ cup almond milk or coconut milk
⅓ cup peeled and sliced orange

1. Line six muffin cups with paper liners.

2. Mix the bananas and milk in a bowl, and then slowly fold in the orange slices. Pour the mixture into the cups.

3. Freeze for at least 1 hour. When it's time to serve, allow the cups to thaw for 10 minutes.

PER SERVING Calories 45   Total carbohydrates 10.6g   Fat 0.3g
Protein 0.9g   Sodium 5mg   Sugar 6.6g

CHOCOLATE FAVE

MAKES 16 SERVINGS   *Prep time: 20 minutes* • *Cook time: 20 minutes*

*Who says you have to give up an old favorite like brownies when you go paleo?
This recipe proves that they are still possible.*

1 cup dates

1 cup walnuts

½ cup raisins

1 banana, mashed

1 teaspoon vanilla extract

½ cup cocoa powder

4 tablespoons coconut flour*

1 tablespoon baking powder

3 eggs

1. Preheat the oven to 350°F.

2. Place the dates, walnuts, and raisins in a food processor, and pulse until finely chopped.

3. Transfer the mixture to a large bowl, add the remaining ingredients, and mix until it becomes a thick, sticky paste.

4. Line an 8-by-8-inch baking pan with parchment paper, and fill with the batter.

5. Bake for 20 minutes. Cool, cut into 16 squares, and serve.

PER SERVING   Calories 114.5   Total carbohydrates 15g   Fat 6.1g
Protein 3.2g   Sodium 82.8mg   Sugar 9.7g

*See page 9 for quick ingredient substitutes and online retailer information

COOKIE TIME

MAKES 24 SERVINGS   *Prep time: 10 minutes • Cook time: 15 minutes*

Paleo, schmaleo—everyone needs a cookie now and then, especially after school or on rainy weekend afternoons. Here is a simple one to make with your kids.

Coconut oil

2 cups unsweetened applesauce

1½ teaspoons baking soda

3 cups almond flour*

½ cup honey

½ cup chopped pecans

½ cup dried cranberries

2 eggs, beaten

¼ cup coconut flour*

2 teaspoons ground cinnamon

2 teaspoons cake spice*

1. Preheat the oven to 400°F.

2. Line two baking sheets with parchment paper and lightly grease with the oil.

3. In a large bowl, stir the applesauce and baking soda until the soda dissolves. Mix in the almond flour, honey, pecans, cranberries, eggs, coconut flour, cinnamon, and cake spice.

4. Drop spoonfuls of the dough 2 inches apart onto the baking sheets.

5. Bake for 15 minutes, checking often for doneness. Cool on a cookie rack and serve warm.

PER SERVING Calories 268   Total carbohydrates 6g   Fat 27g
Protein 6g   Sodium 140g   Sugar 0g

See page 9 for quick ingredient substitutes and online retailer information

HONEY B'S

MAKES 12 SERVINGS   *Prep time: 20 minutes* • *Cook time: 1 hour*

These sweet and crunchy treats are just right for after school or a weekend outing. The honey-almond flavor plus egg protein makes this recipe a winner.

6 eggs
1 cup honey
3½ cups finely ground almonds*
3 teaspoons almond extract

1. Preheat the oven to 300°F.

2. Line a 9-by-9-inch baking pan with parchment paper, and then grease the paper.

3. Using two medium bowls, separate the egg yolks and whites. Beat the yolks until they are quite thick. Add the honey slowly, and then slowly fold in the nuts and extract. Beat the egg whites until they are stiff and fold them into the yolk mix.

4. Pour the batter into the pan and bake for 1 hour.

5. Let it cool for 10 minutes before removing from the pan. Allow to cool completely, and then cut into 12 pieces.

PER SERVING   Calories 375   Total carbohydrates 33.4g   Fat 23.5g
Protein 12g   Sodium 35mg   Sugar 29.1g

*See page 9 for quick ingredient substitutes and online retailer information

GRILLED FRUIT KABOBS

MAKES 8 SERVINGS   *Prep time: 15 minutes • Cook time: 5 minutes*

It's easy enough to get kids to eat an apple or a pear, but if you want to give them something special, this recipe is just the ticket. Oven grilling brings out the natural sweetness of the fruit and caramelizes the honey, making these kabobs extra delicious.

½ teaspoon coconut oil
½ cup fresh pineapple chunks
½ cup fresh watermelon chunks
½ cup fresh cantaloupe chunks
½ cup green seedless grapes
8 bamboo skewers soaked in water for 30 minutes
4 ounces honey
½ teaspoon sea salt

1. Place your oven's broiler rack about 6 inches from the broiler element and turn on the broiler. Line a baking sheet with aluminum foil and grease the foil with coconut oil.

2. Thread the fruits onto the bamboo skewers, alternating them as you like. (Kids love to help with this part.) Lay the skewers in a single layer on the baking sheet.

3. Microwave the honey in a small dish for 15 seconds, then pour it over the fruit skewers. Sprinkle the sea salt over all.

4. Broil for 2 minutes on each side, until just golden. Allow to cool at least 10 minutes before serving, as the fruit will be very hot.

PER SERVING Calories 22   Total carbohydrates 4.6g   Fat 0.4g
Protein 0.3g   Sodium 146.7mg   Sugar 4.3g

5

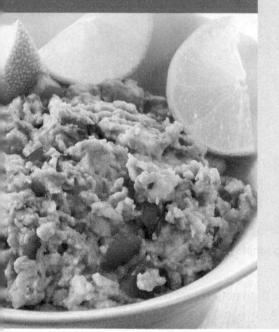

PARTY TIME

The game begins in two hours and everyone is headed to your house to watch, cheer, and, of course, eat! You have an empty table just waiting to be filled with a balance of sweet and salty snacks to please all of your sports fans. What can you make if the usual choices don't fit with your paleo diet? Try these recipes the next time you're the host of the party.

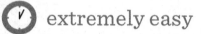 extremely easy

PILES O' PISTACHIOS

If you haven't already discovered the wonder of pistachios, it's time that you do. They're a taste treat that originated in Central Asia and the Middle East. You can buy them already out of the shell, but popping open those shells is part of the enjoyment.

Pistachios typically come roasted and salted, but you can also find them in flavors like chili lemon, habanero, garlic onion, and cilantro lime. They're low in salt and calories, and high in vitamin B_6 and fiber. Put a bowl of them on the table—and watch them disappear.

PER SERVING Calories 691   Total carbohydrates 34g   Fat 56g
Protein 25g   Sodium 1mg   Sugar 0g

OLIVE YOU DIP

MAKES 28 SERVINGS   *Prep time: 20 minutes* • *Cook time: None*

This one is a party favorite and makes enough for lots of guests. It makes use of canned and jarred ingredients, so it's easy to throw together at the last minute.

One 4-ounce can green chiles, chopped
1 onion, chopped
One 5-ounce jar green olives, chopped (reserve liquid)
One 6-ounce can black olives, chopped
1½ cups shredded Cheddar cheese
2 ripe tomatoes, chopped
Black pepper
Garlic salt

1. Put a serving bowl in the freezer to chill while you make this dip.

2. In a large mixing bowl, combine the chiles, onion, and olives. Gently mix in the cheese and then the tomatoes, and season with pepper and garlic salt to taste. Add some of the green olive brine until the mixture is loose but not runny.

3. Transfer the dip to the chilled bowl and serve with crackers or baby carrots.

PER SERVING Calories 42   Total carbohydrates 1.9g   Fat 3.2g
Protein 1.8g   Sodium 253mg   Sugar 0g

MEATZA PIZZA

No gathering seems complete without pizza. Here's a way to make one and stay paleo! It calls for ground beef and pepperoni, plus two kinds of cheese.

1 tablespoon salt	2 eggs
1 teaspoon caraway seeds	½ cup grated Parmesan cheese
1 teaspoon dried oregano	One 12-ounce package shredded
1 teaspoon garlic salt	mozzarella cheese
1 teaspoon black pepper	1 cup tomato sauce
1 teaspoon red pepper flakes	One 3.5-ounce package sliced pepperoni
2 pounds ground beef	

1. Preheat the oven to 450°F.

2. In a small bowl, combine the salt, caraway seeds, oregano, garlic salt, black pepper, and red pepper flakes.

3. In a mixing bowl, mix the ground beef and eggs. Add the Parmesan cheese and the seasoning mixture to it, and combine. Press the mixture into a 12-by-17-inch pan, spreading it out evenly.

4. Bake for about 10 minutes, and then drain the grease. Switch the oven to broil and move the rack to the top position.

5. Sprinkle a third of the mozzarella cheese over the meat, followed by the tomato sauce. Add another third of the cheese and then a layer of pepperoni. Sprinkle the remaining cheese on top.

6. Broil 3 to 5 minutes until the cheese is browned and bubbling.

PER SERVING Calories 506   Total carbohydrates 5.1g   Fat 27.8g
Protein 56.5g   Sodium 252.1mg   Sugar 4g

SAUSAGE BOWLS

MAKES 8 SERVINGS   *Prep time: 10 minutes • Cook time: 30 minutes*

Remember that old favorite, pigs in a blanket? This is the paleo version! You'll need eight ramekins, which are small dishes for baking individual portions of food. You have to start making this dish the night before you want to eat it.

2 pounds ground pork
2 teaspoons salt
2 teaspoons dried sage
1 teaspoon black pepper
⅛ teaspoon ground turmeric
⅛ teaspoon dried marjoram
1 tablespoon butter
8 eggs

1. Preheat the oven to 350°F.

2. Place the pork in a large bowl. In a small bowl, combine the salt, sage, pepper, turmeric, and marjoram. Sprinkle over the pork and stir to combine. Cover with plastic wrap and chill in the refrigerator for at least 8 hours.

3. Butter eight ramekins. Divide the pork mixture into eight balls. Press each one into a ramekin, and create a dip or well in the center. Crack an egg into each dip.

4. Bake 30 to 40 minutes, until the sausage is cooked and the eggs are set.

PER SERVING Calories 318   Total carbohydrates 0.7g   Fat 22.7g
Protein 26.5g   Sodium 719mg   Sugar 0.5g

CRACKLIN' GOOD

MAKES 16 SERVINGS   *Prep time: 30 minutes • Cook time: 20 minutes*

Dip is all well and good, but you need something to dip into the dip. These crackers manage to be paleo and yet tough enough to dip—and double dip.

1 tablespoon coconut oil

4 teaspoons chopped onion

2 garlic cloves, minced

3½ tablespoons chopped fresh
   mushrooms

1 tablespoon frozen chopped spinach,
   thawed and drained

⅓ cup almond flour*

⅓ cup coconut flour*

2 tablespoons flaxseed meal*

½ teaspoon salt

Pinch of black pepper

2 eggs

2 tablespoons water

1 tablespoon olive oil

1. In a skillet over medium heat, melt the oil and then sauté the onion and garlic for 5 minutes. Add the mushrooms and sauté for another 5 minutes. Add the spinach and cook for another 2 to 3 minutes. Remove the pan from the heat and allow the vegetables to cool.

2. Meanwhile, in a large mixing bowl, combine the flours, flaxseed meal, salt, and pepper. Preheat the oven to 350°F.

3. Transfer the cooled vegetable mix to a cutting board and chop finely. Stir the vegetables into the flour mixture; then add the eggs, water, and oil. Mix until it forms a dough.

4. Line a baking sheet with parchment paper and press the dough onto it. Place another piece of parchment paper on top, and roll out the dough until it is about $1/16$ inch thick. Take off the top piece of paper and cut off the edges of the dough to make the edges even. Cut the dough into 1-inch squares.

5. Bake for 18 to 20 minutes, until the edges are browned. Cool for 1 hour and then break into squares.

PER SERVING Calories 66   Total carbohydrates 4.6g   Fat 4.5g
Protein 2.3g   Sodium 82mg   Sugar 2.0g

See page 9 for quick ingredient substitutes and online retailer information

ALMOND TREATS

Need a sweet treat for the snack table? This one is quick and simple to make—and a good source of protein, too. You might want to double or triple this recipe because it goes fast!

2 cups almond flour*
1½ tablespoons warm honey
1½ teaspoons ground cinnamon
½ teaspoon ground nutmeg
3 egg whites

1. Preheat the oven to 350°F.

2. Line a baking sheet with parchment paper.

3. In a large mixing bowl, combine the almond flour, honey, cinnamon, and nutmeg. In a medium mixing bowl, beat the eggs whites until they are stiff, and then combine with the almond mixture.

4. Drop the mixture onto the baking sheet by the teaspoonful, and bake for 10 to 15 minutes, until browned.

PER SERVING   Calories 90   Total carbohydrates 8g   Fat 3.5g
Protein 8.4g   Sodium 15mg   Sugar 7.6g

See page 9 for quick ingredient substitutes and online retailer information

BEAN-FREE CHILI

MAKES 4 SERVINGS   *Prep time: 15 minutes* • *Cook time: 35 minutes*

This chili is smoky and flavorful, but remember you want to make it the day before the game, if possible. It gives the flavors a chance to blend and get friendly. This is a spicy chili, so if you have children coming to the party, make them their own batch without the chipotle pepper and with regular sweet pork sausage.

1 dried chipotle pepper, stem removed

1 cup boiling water

1½ teaspoons coconut oil

1 cup chopped yellow onion

1 cup chopped green bell pepper

1 cup chopped red bell pepper

4 garlic cloves, minced

1 pound ground beef

½ pound spicy ground pork sausage

1 tablespoon chili powder

1 tablespoon ground cumin

1 teaspoon dried oregano

1 teaspoon unsweetened cocoa powder

1 teaspoon Worcestershire sauce

One 28-ounce can crushed tomatoes

1½ teaspoons salt

½ teaspoon black pepper

1. Soak the chipotle pepper in boiling water for 10 minutes, until softened. Remove from the water and mince.

2. In a large pot over medium heat, melt the oil. Stir in the onions and bell peppers and cook 5 to 10 minutes until tender. Add the garlic and the minced chipotle, and cook another 1 to 2 minutes.

3. Stir the two meats into the mixture and cook for 10 to 12 minutes, until the meat is thoroughly browned. Add the spices, cocoa powder, and Worcestershire sauce, as well as the tomatoes, salt, and pepper. Mix thoroughly and bring to a boil.

4. Reduce heat to low and simmer for another 10 minutes. You can eat it now—but if you wait until tomorrow, it will taste even richer.

PER SERVING Calories 380   Total carbohydrates 26.4g   Fat 17.2g
Protein 33g   Sodium 1,567mg   Sugar 18.6g

HOLY GUACAMOLE!

MAKES 6 SERVINGS   *Prep time: 15 minutes • Cook time: None*

Pork rinds, paleo crackers, and raw veggies always taste good dipped in guacamole. Forget the store-bought kind with its preservatives and other unnecessary ingredients, and make your own. If you don't care for spicy foods, skip the jalapeño.

2 ripe avocados, peeled and pitted

1 lime, juiced

1 jalapeño pepper, diced

1 clove garlic, minced

½ small onion, minced

1 Roma tomato, seeded and diced

1 tablespoon chopped fresh cilantro

Salt and pepper

1. Place the avocados in a medium serving bowl, and squeeze the lime juice on top of them.

2. Using a fork, smash the avocados and then add the remaining ingredients. Combine with a fork, and serve.

PER SERVING Calories 118   Total carbohydrates 8.2g   Fat 9.9g
Protein 1.7g   Sodium 71mg   Sugar 7.2g

CRAB FEST

MAKES 6 SERVINGS   *Prep time: 15 minutes*   •   *Cook time: 20 minutes*

Your party guests who are seafood lovers will enjoy this dish! Fresh crabmeat is always a terrific treat, and the Worcestershire and hot sauces kick it up a notch.

1 large egg

2 tablespoons mayonnaise

1 teaspoon Dijon mustard

½ teaspoon Worcestershire sauce

¼ teaspoon hot pepper sauce

¼ teaspoon lemon juice

½ teaspoon seafood seasoning

Black pepper

1 pound fresh lump crabmeat

¼ cup plus ⅓ cup almond flour*

1 tablespoon finely diced red pepper

2 tablespoons sliced green onion

1 tablespoon chopped fresh parsley

1. Grease a baking sheet. In a medium bowl, whisk together the egg, mayonnaise, mustard, Worcestershire sauce, hot sauce, lemon juice, seasoning, and pepper.

2. Place the crabmeat in a large bowl and pour the mixture over it. Using your hands, combine thoroughly. Mix in ¼ cup almond flour, red pepper, green onion, and parsley.

3. Form the mixture into six patties. Place the remaining ⅓ cup almond flour in a shallow bowl. Put each patty in the flour and cover each side thoroughly. When all patties are done, place them on the baking sheet and chill them in the refrigerator for an hour or more.

4. When the time is up, preheat the oven to 400°F. Bake the crab cakes for 15 to 20 minutes until golden brown.

PER SERVING Calories 177   Total carbohydrates 4.8g   Fat 7.5g
Protein 22.4g   Sodium 488mg   Sugar 4.6g

*See page 9 for quick ingredient substitutes and online retailer information

IT'S A WRAP!

MAKES 4 SERVINGS   *Prep time: 20 minutes* • *Cook time: 35 minutes*

Wraps are ideal snacks for people to grab with their hands—because who needs plates at a party? These wraps are incredibly rich in texture and flavor.

2 boneless, skinless chicken breasts, split in half lengthwise
8 ounces crumbled blue cheese
3 ounces walnut halves
3 ounces pecan halves
8 slices bacon

1. Preheat the oven to 350°F.

2. Pound the chicken breasts halves until they are about ¼ inch thick. Arrange the blue cheese, walnuts, and pecans on top of each chicken piece, and then roll them up.

3. Put the bacon slices side by side on a cutting board or other work surface. Place each chicken roll at one end of two slices and roll the bacon around the chicken. Secure it in place with toothpicks. Repeat with each of the rolls.

4. In a skillet over medium heat, cook the bacon-wrapped chicken rolls until the bacon is crisp, about 4 to 5 minutes per side.

5. Transfer the rolls to the oven and bake for 25 to 35 minutes, until the chicken is no longer pink in the center.

PER SERVING Calories 637   Total carbohydrates 7.4g   Fat 52.8g
Protein 36.8g   Sodium 1,238mg   Sugar 4.8g

KICK IT BBQ SAUCE

MAKES 8 SERVINGS   *Prep time: 15 minutes* • *Cook time: 20 minutes*

This is a great sauce to add to any meat you're serving, plus it can be added to egg dishes or even stand alone as a thick, spicy dip. Best of all, it's easy!

1 cup beef stock

One 6-ounce can tomato paste

¼ cup minced shallots

1 tablespoon Dijon mustard

3 garlic cloves, minced

2 tablespoons apple cider vinegar

1 teaspoon ground cumin

1 teaspoon cayenne pepper

1 teaspoon black pepper

1 teaspoon prepared horseradish

1 teaspoon red pepper flakes

½ teaspoon salt

1. Put all the ingredients in a saucepan over medium heat. Bring to a simmer, stirring until well combined.

2. Reduce heat to medium-low, cover, and simmer for 15 to 20 minutes, until the sauce thickens a little. Be sure to stir often.

PER SERVING   Calories 60   Total carbohydrates 6.8g   Fat 2.2g
Protein 1.8g   Sodium 375mg   Sugar 5.5g

SALMON BITES

MAKES 4 SERVINGS   *Prep time: 10 minutes* • *Cook time: 10 minutes*

A delight for the seafood fans at your house. Wild Alaskan salmon packs those good-for-you omega-3 fatty acids, and there's plenty of protein here, too.

One 7.5-ounce can wild Alaskan salmon
¼ cup almond meal*
3 eggs
2 tablespoons olive oil
Salt and pepper

1. In a large bowl, mix the salmon, almond meal, eggs, and 1 tablespoon oil. Season with salt and pepper.

2. Form the mixture into patties, about ½ cup per patty.

3. In a skillet over medium heat, heat the remaining 1 tablespoon oil and cook the patties for about 5 minutes per side, until browned.

PER SERVING Calories 231   Total carbohydrates 2.3g   Fat 15.7g
Protein 19.9g   Sodium 342mg   Sugar 2.0g

* See page 9 for quick ingredient substitutes and online retailer information

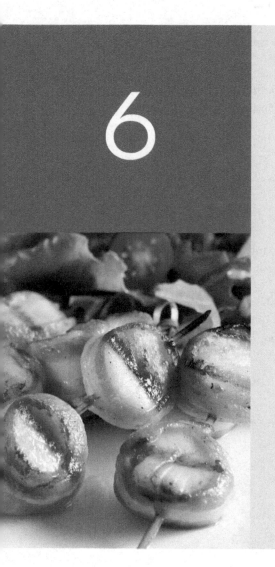

6

PROTEIN PERFECTION

On the paleo diet, getting enough protein into your meals is rarely a problem. With an emphasis on meat and eggs, the grams add up quickly. However, if you're concerned that your numbers are low, or if you don't have time for an entire meal and want to have a snack that's packed with protein, here's a chapter full of great dishes—with some exotic ingredients—to give you a boost.

A few of these recipes help you get your protein by drinking it. They rely on stevia to give them a naturally sweet taste, and unsweetened gelatin powder, which is good for your cardiovascular system, to add texture.

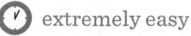

TOPPED APPLES

Consider the apple—it's a perfectly packaged bundle of nutrition. The average large apple has about 115 calories, plus 5 grams of fiber and enough vitamin C to fulfill about 18 percent of your daily requirements. Apples come in all different colors and flavors, and best of all, they can be topped with a wide variety of paleo ingredients that make this fruit taste even better.

Try these topping ideas for your sliced apple:

- Sprinkles of cinnamon
- Shredded, melted cheese
- Tahini
- Almond butter or cashew butter
- Slivered almonds
- Chopped pecans or walnuts

BANANA NUT CEREAL

MAKES 2 SERVINGS   *Prep time: 5 minutes* • *Cook time: 5 minutes*

There's no reason hot cereal should be eaten only for breakfast. It makes a great snack, too! This paleo version is filling and satisfying.

½ cup almonds, whole or slivered
½ cup pecans
½ banana
¼ teaspoon ground cinnamon
¼ teaspoon salt
¼ cup unsweetened almond or coconut milk
Handful of nuts or fresh berries of your choice for garnish

1. Place all ingredients in a food processor, and pulse until the texture is as chunky or smooth as you prefer.

2. Heat the cereal in the microwave or on the stove until it is hot. Garnish with more nuts or some fresh berries, if available.

PER SERVING Calories 487   Total carbohydrates 19g   Fat 45g
Protein 11g   Sodium 2mg   Sugar 0g

EGG BURRITO

MAKES 2 SERVINGS   *Prep time: 5 minutes • Cook time: 20 minutes*

Who doesn't enjoy a burrito on the go? But how do you make one without a tortilla? Here's how! It's also a perfect way to use up that leftover ground beef, steak, or chicken in the refrigerator.

4 eggs, whites and yolks separated

½ onion, finely chopped

Olive oil

2 tomatoes, finely chopped

¼ cup canned diced green chiles

1 red pepper, cut into strips

¼ cup finely chopped cilantro

½ cup cooked meat of your choice

1 avocado, chunked

½ cup salsa or dash of hot sauce

1. Using two bowls, separate the whites and the yolks, and whisk the whites together. Pour half of the egg whites in a skillet over low heat, moving the pan in circles to ensure the whites are spread evenly and thinly across the surface. After 30 seconds, cover and cook for another minute. This is your tortilla! Gently slide it out of the pan with a spatula and repeat for a second tortilla.

2. Sauté the onion in oil for 1 to 2 minutes, and then add the tomatoes, green chiles, red pepper, cilantro, and cooked meat.

3. Whisk the egg yolks together, and pour them into the pan with the meat and vegetables to create a scramble. Stir until cooked.

4. Divide the filling between the tortillas, and add the avocado chunks and salsa. Roll up and eat!

PER SERVING Calories 524   Total carbohydrates 30g   Fat 35g
Protein 27g   Sodium (varies according to meat used)   Sugar 4g

SPICY EGGS

MAKES 2 SERVINGS   *Prep time: 5 minutes* • *Cook time: 15 minutes*

As you know, eggs manage to hold an amazing amount of protein inside those shells. This dish is easy to make, and so fast!

4 slices bacon

6 eggs

1 teaspoon horseradish

1. Cut the bacon into small pieces and fry it in a large skillet until crisp. Remove the bacon and set aside. Leave 1 tablespoon of bacon drippings in the skillet.

2. In a medium mixing bowl, whisk the eggs together with the horseradish. Pour the eggs into the hot bacon drippings, and scramble in the skillet over medium heat. Just before the eggs are completely set, add the bacon back in and scramble to combine.

PER SERVING   Calories 450   Total carbohydrates 2g   Fat 34g
Protein 20g   Sodium 23mg   Sugar 0g

HOT GREENS

Prep time: 5 minutes • Cook time: 10 minutes

Salads are healthy snacks that can usually be made quickly. Here is a twist that adds protein along with a truly gourmet taste. Putting fried eggs on top just makes it even better.

1 small head of arugula or frisée
1 small head of romaine or 2 large handfuls of fresh spinach
½ pound bacon, cut into small pieces
1 shallot, finely chopped
3 tablespoons sherry vinegar
1 tablespoon mustard
2 eggs

1. Tear the greens into bite-size pieces and put in a salad bowl.

2. In a skillet over medium heat, sauté the bacon until crisp, and then add the shallot. Sauté for a few more minutes, and then add the vinegar and mustard. Stir as it boils for 20 to 30 seconds, and then remove from the heat. While still hot, pour the mixture over the greens. They will wilt a bit—and taste amazing.

3. In a skillet over medium heat, fry the eggs in oil and then place on top of the salad.

PER SERVING Calories 422   Total carbohydrates 9g   Fat 29g
Protein 30g   Sodium 58mg   Sugar 11g

TUNABERRY SALAD

MAKES 2 SERVINGS   *Prep time: 10 minutes • Cook time: None*

If you like foods with a great deal of texture, this is the salad for you. It's ready in only a matter of minutes and packs more than 40 grams of protein per serving. Eat it as is or put on a bed of greens if time and appetite allow.

12 ounces canned tuna

2 celery stalks, finely chopped

¼ cup finely chopped red onion

¼ cup mayonnaise

½ cup dried cranberries

Mix all ingredients together in a bowl and serve.

PER SERVING Calories 487   Total carbohydrates 27g   Fat 23g
Protein 43g   Sodium 640mg   Sugar 15g

SIMMERIN' SHRIMP SOUP

MAKES 3 SERVINGS   *Prep time: 5 minutes • Cook time: 10 minutes*

Hot soup makes one of the best possible snacks, especially on chilly days and nights. Coconut milk is used as a base, and the shrimp loads it full of protein.

Two 15-ounce cans coconut milk
Few handfuls of fresh spinach
1 tablespoon butter
1 pound raw shrimp, peeled and deveined
1½ tablespoons curry powder
Salt

1. In a blender, purée the coconut milk and spinach until smooth.

2. In a pot on the stove over medium-high heat, melt the butter and then add the shrimp and curry powder. Sauté for 2 minutes and then add the spinach mixture. Bring to a boil, and then turn off the heat. Add salt to taste, and serve.

PER SERVING Calories 529   Total carbohydrates 10g   Fat 36g
Protein 46g   Sodium 1,341mg   Sugar 16g

BACON SCALLOPS

MAKES 3 SERVINGS   *Prep time: 10 minutes* • *Cook time: 10 minutes*

This recipe is a fabulous blend of contasting flavors and textures. Feel like treating yourself? This is the dish to make.

4 slices of bacon
½ cup almonds
1 large handful of parsley
1 pound scallops

1. In a skillet over medium heat, cook the bacon until crispy enough to easily crumble. Crumble and set aside, leaving the bacon drippings in the pan.

2. Place the almonds, parsley, and bacon in a food processor, and pulse until everything is in small pieces.

3. Add the scallops to the skillet with the leftover bacon drippings, and turn the heat to high. Cook for 2 minutes until the scallops are browned on one side, and then flip them over and cook the other side for 1 to 2 minutes.

4. Transfer the scallops to a plate and sprinkle the bacon-nut mix over the top.

PER SERVING   Calories 413   Total carbohydrates 10g   Fat 28g
Protein 33g   Sodium 955mg   Sugar 1g

WALNUT PROTEIN SAUCE

MAKES 1 CUP   *Prep time: 5 minutes • Cook time: 10 minutes*

One way to increase your protein intake is through the addition of a higher protein sauce like this one. It can be added to steamed veggies or to meat for extra flavor.

2 tablespoons butter
1 cup walnuts
1 shallot, finely chopped
1½ cups heavy cream or coconut milk
Salt

1. In a large skillet over medium heat, melt the butter and sauté the walnuts and shallot until the nuts are lightly toasted, about 3 minutes.

2. Add 1 cup cream, season with salt, and simmer lightly for 5 minutes.

3. Pour the mixture into a blender and purée until smooth. If the sauce is too thick, add the remaining cream.

PER SERVING Calories 244   Total carbohydrates 6g   Fat 24g
Protein 5g   Sodium 0.5mg   Sugar 0mg

MEXISMOOTH

MAKES 1 SERVING   *Prep time: 5 minutes • Cook time: None*

Mexican cooking is known for combining chocolate and cinnamon, such as in this rich drink. It takes only minutes to make and will keep you full for hours.

½ cup unsweetened coconut milk, chilled

2 eggs

4 teaspoons cocoa powder

¾ teaspoon French vanilla liquid stevia*

½ teaspoon ground cinnamon

½ teaspoon unsweetened gelatin powder

1. Place all ingredients in a blender.

2. Blend until smooth. Pour and enjoy!

PER SERVING Calories 376   Total carbohydrates 9g   Fat 33g
Protein 16g   Sodium 13mg   Sugar 4g

* See page 9 for quick ingredient substitutes and online retailer information

COCONOG

MAKES 1 SERVING   *Prep time: 5 minutes*   •   *Cook time: None*

Why wait for the holidays for these delicious flavors? This smoothie is super simple and contains 15 grams of protein per serving.

1 cup unsweetened coconut milk

2 eggs

15 drops French vanilla liquid stevia*

1 teaspoon vanilla extract

¼ teaspoon ground nutmeg

¼ teaspoon ground cinnamon

1. Place all ingredients in a blender.

2. Blend until smooth. Pour and enjoy!

PER SERVING   Calories 590   Total carbohydrates 9g   Fat 56g
Protein 15g   Sodium 13mg   Sugar 0g

*See page 9 for quick ingredient substitutes and online retailer information

STRAWBERRY BLISS

MAKES 1 SERVING   *Prep time: 5 minutes* • *Cook time: None*

Although this is technically a smoothie, it's thick enough to eat with a spoon. The frozen strawberries and the gelatin powder give it that appealing dense consistency.

8 strawberries, frozen
½ cup unsweetened coconut milk
2 eggs
1 teaspoon lemon juice
10 drops liquid stevia*
½ teaspoon unflavored gelatin powder

1. Place all ingredients in a blender.

2. Blend until smooth. If it's too thick, add a little water to reach your desired consistency. Pour and enjoy!

PER SERVING   Calories 376   Total carbohydrates 9g   Fat 33g
Protein 14g   Sodium 13mg   Sugar 5g

*See page 9 for quick ingredient substitutes and online retailer information

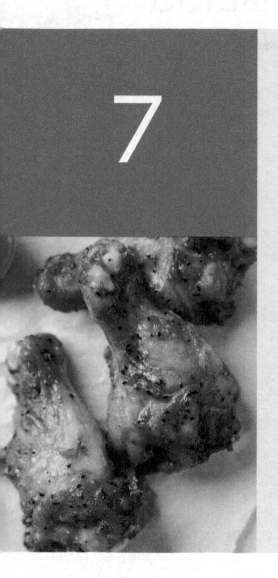

7

CALLING ALL MEAT LOVERS

Anyone who decides to follow the paleo lifestyle has to really like meat, as it is an essential part of the diet. Finding high-quality meat is critical, so start by seeking out local butchers and organic, grass-fed sources.

All of the snacks in this chapter incorporate meat to provide quick, high-protein mini meals. From pork to turkey, beef, bacon, and chicken, there's something here for everyone in your household.

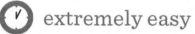

PORK RINDS ITALIANO

If there's one food that brings the word *unhealthy* to mind, it has to be pork rinds. However, they really don't deserve that reputation. Pork rinds are one of the healthiest snacks out there and can be just what you need when you're hankering for that special crunch. They contain quite a bit of gelatin, which is good for your joints, nails, and hair. Gelatin is also an anti-inflammatory.

To jazz up basic store-bought pork rinds, open the bag and add ½ teaspoon dried parsley, ½ teaspoon oregano, ¼ teaspoon garlic, and ¼ teaspoon onion powder. Close the bag, shake it up, and then try the seasoned pork rinds.

JUMPIN' JERKY

MAKES 5 SERVINGS   *Prep time: 10 minutes • Cook time: 5 to 6 hours*

There's a reason jerky has been around for decades—it's part of American history. It's full of protein and other nutritional value, and can keep well in the refrigerator for ages. This recipe for jerky is also full of spice and heat! It takes a while to prepare and bake, so don't be in a hurry. The time and effort are worth it.

⅔ cup soy sauce

⅓ cup hot water

¼ cup Worcestershire sauce

1 tablespoon liquid smoke flavoring

1 tablespoon onion powder

1½ teaspoons cayenne pepper

1½ teaspoons Creole-style seasoning

1½ teaspoons Cajun seasoning blend

2½ pounds London broil sliced roast beef

1. In a medium microwave-safe bowl, whisk together all of the ingredients except the roast beef. Microwave on high for 1 minute.

2. Stir and then add the slices of meat, making sure each one is coated on both sides. Cover the bowl and marinate the meat in the refrigerator overnight.

3. The next day, preheat the oven to 160°F. Once you take the meat out of the marinade, rinse it with hot water. Place the meat strips on a rack about an inch apart from each other.

4. Bake in the oven for 5 to 6 hours. Allow to cool.

PER SERVING Calories 68   Total carbohydrates 8.5g   Fat 2.9g
Protein 2.7g   Sodium 2,344mg   Sugar 0mg

SAUSAGE STYLE

MAKES 8 SERVINGS   *Prep time: 20 minutes* • *Cook time: 20 minutes*

Sausage isn't just for breakfast anymore. These patties are so good, they work for any meal, as well as a high-protein snack. The spices make these especially tasty.

1 pound ground pork

1 teaspoon salt

¾ teaspoon black pepper

2 teaspoons finely chopped fresh
   sage leaves

1 teaspoon finely chopped fresh thyme

¼ teaspoon chopped fresh rosemary

¼ teaspoon ground nutmeg

¼ teaspoon ground cloves

½ teaspoon fennel seeds

¼ teaspoon cayenne pepper

¼ teaspoon red pepper flakes

1. In a medium bowl, mix all ingredients together, using your hands to make sure it is well combined.

2. Form into eight patties and place in a skillet over medium heat. Cook 8 to 10 minutes until browned. Flip and continue to cook until the other side is brown, about 5 to 8 minutes.

PER SERVING Calories 118   Total carbohydrates 12.7g   Fat 8.2g
Protein 10.1g   Sodium 269mg   Sugar 0.2g

TURKEY TREAT

Want to try a new spin on chili? This one not only doesn't use beans—it doesn't use any tomatoes, and it does use pumpkin seeds. What a combination! Although any heavy kettle will do, a Dutch oven definitely works best.

3 pounds ground turkey

¼ cup olive oil

1 quart unsalted chicken broth

6 tablespoons chili powder

10 garlic cloves, crushed

½ teaspoon ground cumin

1 teaspoon dried oregano

1 teaspoon cayenne pepper

½ teaspoon black pepper

1 tablespoon unsweetened cocoa powder

2 teaspoons honey

3 tablespoons paprika

½ cup shelled pumpkin seeds

Salt

1. In the Dutch oven, brown the turkey in the oil. Once the meat is no longer pink, add the broth, chili powder, garlic, cumin, oregano, cayenne pepper, black pepper, cocoa powder, honey, and paprika. Bring to a simmer and cook for 1 hour.

2. While the mixture is simmering, run the pumpkin seeds through the food processor until finely ground, like cornmeal.

3. At the end of the hour, stir in the ground pumpkin seeds and simmer for another 15 to 20 minutes. Season with salt.

PER SERVING   Calories 522   Total carbohydrates 13g   Fat 31g
Protein 49g   Sodium 233mg   Sugar 2.5g

ROAST AND WINE

MAKES 2 SERVINGS   *Prep time: 30 minutes* • *Cook time: 30 minutes*

Roast and wine—truly a wonderful blend of flavors. Although this recipe uses beef roast, you can substitute whatever kind of meat you prefer. Make a few batches and then divide up for between-meal snacks.

1 pound roast, cubed

1 cup wine (red if beef, white if other meat)

⅓ cup finely diced onion

1 cup finely chopped mushrooms

½ cup finely diced carrots

3 tablespoons olive oil

1 teaspoon dried thyme

1 teaspoon dried oregano

⅛ teaspoon black pepper

1. In a large skillet, sauté the roast, wine, onion, mushrooms, and carrots in the oil until the meat is browned and the vegetables have softened.

2. Turn the heat down and add the spices. Simmer for another 15 minutes, stirring occasionally.

PER SERVING Calories 720   Total carbohydrates 9.7g   Fat 39.5g
Protein 62.4g   Sodium 153mg   Sugar 3.7g

POTATO SALAD PALEO

MAKES 1 SERVING   *Prep time: 5 minutes • Cook time: 20 minutes*

Did you think potato salad was a part of your past? It doesn't have to be if you use sweet potatoes instead. Here's a recipe that even adds an extra flavor—bacon! This makes enough for one large serving or two side servings. Chances are you'll want to double or triple it.

2 eggs
2/3 cup diced sweet potato
2 slices bacon, diced
1 tablespoon fresh dill, finely chopped
2 tablespoons mayonnaise
2 tablespoons lemon juice

1. In a large pot, boil the eggs in water for 4 to 6 minutes and then drain, peel, and dice them.

2. In a large pot, boil the sweet potato for 4 to 5 minutes until cooked through.

3. In a skillet over medium heat, fry the bacon until browned and crunchy.

4. In a medium bowl, combine the dill, mayonnaise, and lemon juice. Add the eggs, sweet potato, and bacon, and mix well.

PER SERVING Calories 537   Total carbohydrates 44g   Fat 33.3g
Protein 19.8g   Sodium 413mg   Sugar 11.9g

STIR-FRY BEEF

MAKES 2 SERVINGS   *Prep time: 20 minutes • Cook time: 10 minutes*

A stir-fry is always a great way to make a quick and nutritious snack. Sirloin steak and burgundy wine make this one special.

12 ounces sirloin steak, thinly sliced

2 tablespoons olive oil

1 garlic clove, pressed

¼ cup burgundy wine

1 onion, chopped

2 celery stalks, chopped

1 red pepper, seeded and cut into strips

4 ounces carrots, chopped

4 ounces mushrooms, sliced

3 tablespoons lemon juice

1. In a large skillet, sauté the steak in a tablespoon of oil with the garlic and half of the wine until the meat is browned. Remove the meat from the skillet and heat the other tablespoon of oil, adding the onion, celery, red pepper, and carrots. Cook for 4 to 6 minutes until tender.

2. Add the rest of the wine, and then add the mushrooms and lemon juice. Stir-fry the vegetables for another 3 to 5 minutes.

3. Add the meat back in, stir, and heat through.

PER SERVING Calories 548   Total carbohydrates 20.3g   Fat 25.1g
Protein 55.4g   Sodium 173mg   Sugar 9.4g

DEVILED EGGS AND BACON

MAKES 12 SERVINGS   *Prep time: 20 minutes • Cook time: 15 minutes*

Anyone can make deviled eggs, but most are run of the mill. These are distinctive—they combine flavors like bacon and celery salt that make them stand out.

6 eggs

2 slices bacon

3 tablespoons mayonnaise

½ teaspoon celery salt

2 tablespoons minced red onion

¼ teaspoon black pepper

½ teaspoon balsamic vinegar

½ teaspoon brown mustard

Minced fresh parsley for garnish

1. In a large pot, boil the eggs in water until hard-boiled, about 15 minutes. While the eggs are boiling, fry the bacon in a skillet over medium heat. Drain and set aside.

2. When the eggs are done, peel and halve them, removing the yolks and transferring them to a medium mixing bowl. Set the whites aside.

3. Add the mayonnaise to the yolks and mash together until thoroughly mixed. Crumble the bacon into it; then add the celery salt, red onion, pepper, balsamic vinegar, and mustard. Mix until well combined.

4. Scoop the yolk mixture into the halved whites. Sprinkle with the parsley and serve.

PER SERVING Calories 71   Total carbohydrates 1g   Fat 6g
Protein 4g   Sodium 58.8mg   Sugar 1g

WINGIN' IT

MAKES 20 SERVINGS   *Prep time: 15 minutes • Cook time: 45 minutes*

What says "snack" better than chicken wings? There are many paleo wing recipes out there, but here is one of the best and easiest. Omit the hot sauce if you don't like it spicy.

2 pounds chicken wings

¼ cup olive oil

Juice of 1 lemon

2 tablespoons brown mustard

2 garlic cloves, crushed

¼ teaspoon black pepper

¼ teaspoon hot sauce

1. Cut the wings at the joints, and put all of them into a ziplock plastic bag.

2. In a small bowl, mix all of the remaining ingredients and pour over the wings. Seal the bag and turn it to make sure all of the wings are coated. Chill in the refrigerator for 2 hours.

3. Preheat the oven to 375°F. Place the wings on a baking sheet, reserving the marinade left in the bag.

4. Bake the wings for 45 minutes, making sure to pull them out twice to add more marinade. During the last 20 minutes of baking, add the last of the marinade.

PER SERVING Calories 81   Total carbohydrates 1g   Fat 7g
Protein 5g   Sodium 24mg   Sugar 0g

CRAB AND CUKES

MAKES 1 CUP   *Prep time: 10 minutes* • *Cook time: None*

If your idea of a meat lover's dish comes from the sea, you'll enjoy this recipe. And talk about easy! The cucumber slices are perfect for scooping up the spicy crabmeat.

1 teaspoon tomato paste

¼ cup mayonnaise

1 tablespoon chopped chives

1 teaspoon lemon juice

1 teaspoon horseradish

Dash of hot sauce

½ pound crabmeat

1 large cucumber, sliced in rounds

1. In a medium bowl, whisk together the tomato paste, mayonnaise, chives, lemon juice, horseradish, and hot sauce.

2. Add the crabmeat and mix well. Serve with a bowl of sliced cucumber.

PER SERVING   Calories 109   Total carbohydrates 1g   Fat 8g
Protein 8g   Sodium 55mg   Sugar 0g

BACON BUNDLES

MAKES 4 SERVINGS   *Prep time: 5 minutes* • *Cook time: 10 minutes*

Ready for an influx of vitamins A and B, plus iron, copper, and folic acid? Make this snack and it will make your taste buds—and your cardiovascular system—grateful.

1 pound chicken livers
Olive oil
One 12-ounce package of bacon

1. Cut up the chicken livers so that they are about the same length and size. In a large skillet over medium heat, cook them in a little oil, 2 minutes per side.

2. After they are done and cooling, wrap each one in a slice of bacon. Try to cover all of the liver firmly so there is less chance the bacon will fall off.

3. Put the livers back into the skillet, and cook over medium heat for about 3 minutes per side.

PER SERVING   Calories 648   Total carbohydrates 2g   Fat 43g
Protein 59g   Sodium 24g   Sugar 0g

COCONUT CURRY CHICKEN

MAKES 6 SERVINGS   *Prep time: 20 minutes • Cook time: 15 minutes*

Despite what your kids might think, meatballs aren't just for spaghetti anymore—and you don't need breadcrumbs to make this version. It uses freshly ground chicken and complements it with curry and coconut.

1½ pounds boneless, skinless chicken (thighs, breasts, or a combination)
1 carrot, grated
2 garlic cloves
½ cup shredded coconut
1 egg
2 teaspoons curry powder
Handful of cilantro
Olive oil

1. Place all of the ingredients except the oil in a food processor, and pulse until smooth. Transfer the mixture to a large bowl.

2. Form 24 meatballs (your hands will work best for this task), about the size of a golf ball.

3. Heat the oil in a skillet over medium-high heat, and add all of the meatballs as soon as the oil is very hot. Cook for 2 minutes; then roll them over and cook for another 5 minutes. Cover the skillet and cook for another 6 to 8 minutes.

PER SERVING Calories 260   Total carbohydrates 4g   Fat 11g
Protein 34g   Sodium 0g   Sugar 0g

DIPPING CHICKEN

MAKES 3 SERVINGS   *Prep time: 10 minutes* • *Cook time: 10 minutes*

Missing chicken strips from the deli? Here's how to have them in a much healthier way and with an amazingly delicious dipping sauce with an Asian flair.

For the chicken:

1½ pounds chicken breasts,
  cut into thin strips

3 tablespoons tamari

1 tablespoon sesame oil

2 teaspoons ground coriander

1 teaspoon ground cumin

For the dipping sauce:

½ cup almond flour*

¼ cup coconut milk

¼ cup water

1 garlic clove

2 teaspoons ginger, minced

1 teaspoon tamari

3 teaspoons sesame oil

1½ tablespoons fish sauce

1. Heat the oven to broil.

2. Place the chicken in a large bowl and season with the tamari, sesame oil, coriander, and cumin. Broil for 10 minutes.

3. Meanwhile, put all of the ingredients for the sauce into a food processor and process until smooth. Serve the sauce with the chicken.

PER SERVING   Calories 760   Total carbohydrates 12g   Fat 45g
Protein 79g   Sodium 879mg   Sugar 0g

*See page 9 for quick ingredient substitutes and online retailer information

THE BEST BCLTA

MAKES 1 SERVING   *Prep time: 5 minutes • Cook time: 20 minutes*

This takes a little more effort to make, but when you're craving an excellent sandwich, this bacon-chicken-lettuce-tomato-avocado recipe is guaranteed to hit the spot. Who needs bread, anyway? This makes one serving, so be prepared to double (or triple) it, share it, or make it only when no one else is home.

1 chicken breast

Salt and pepper

Olive oil

1 tablespoon mayonnaise

2 slices cooked bacon

2 to 3 leaves romaine lettuce

1 tomato, thinly sliced

1 avocado, thinly sliced

1. Cut the chicken breast nearly in half lengthwise without cutting all the way through, and lightly season with salt and pepper. Open up the chicken breast, and in a medium skillet, sear it in hot oil for 4 to 6 minutes on the first side. Flip it and do the same for the other side. Depending on the thickness of the chicken, this will take another 6 to 10 minutes.

2. Remove the chicken and spread mayonnaise on one side. Layer on the bacon, lettuce, tomato, and avocado, and then close the chicken breast. Voilá—a sandwich!

PER SERVING Calories 878   Total carbohydrates 22g   Fat 60g
Protein 67g   Sodium 45mg   Sugar 1g

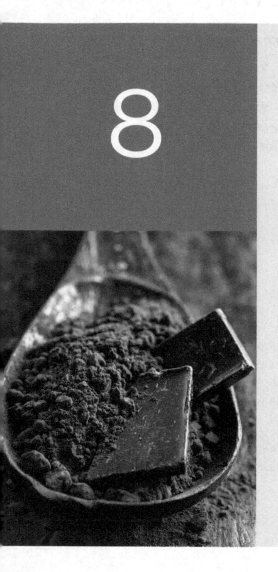

8

A SWEET TREAT

Chances are if you've been on the paleo diet for a while, your sweet tooth has shifted to a lower gear. (And if you're just starting out, be patient—it will change over time.) What once tasted great now tastes far too sweet. Dishes made with regular white and brown sugars can be intense. Anything less than 70 percent chocolate isn't as rich and satisfying as the darker choices.

Paleo relies on a few sweeteners like agave and stevia, but for the most part, it obtains its sweet flavors through more natural options such as dates and fruit, as well as maple syrup and honey. As your palate adjusts to the paleo lifestyle, the sweet snacks in this chapter will taste better and better.

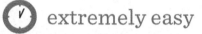

HERBED WATERMELON

MAKES 12 SERVINGS · *Prep time: 20 minutes* · *Cook time: None*

How can you possibly improve on the fresh, sweet taste of watermelon? You can't—but you can include it in this recipe for a new take on a favorite flavor. The ingredients list may be a bit long, but the preparation is a snap.

½ large chilled seedless watermelon, cut into 1-inch cubes

1 small red onion, sliced

1 cup thinly sliced fresh basil leaves

1 cup chopped fresh cilantro

½ cup minced fresh mint leaves

Juice of 2 limes

4 ounces crumbled feta cheese (optional)

3 tablespoons olive oil

2 tablespoons balsamic vinegar

Salt and pepper

1. Place the first nine ingredients in a large bowl.

2. Season with salt and pepper, and gently mix. It's ready to go!

PER SERVING Calories 177 Total carbohydrates 31.1g Fat 6g
Protein 4g Sodium 144mg Sugar 29g

CHOCOLATE ZUCCHINI BARS

MAKES 3 SERVINGS   *Prep time: 25 minutes* • *Cook time: 50 to 60 minutes*

Life without brownies is too sad to think about, so here is a paleo version of this much beloved treat. Applesauce and honey provide the sweetness.

3 eggs
½ cup honey
3 tablespoons olive oil
¾ cup applesauce
1 cup almond meal*
¼ cup cocoa powder
½ teaspoon baking powder
½ cup walnuts, chopped
2 cups grated zucchini

1. Preheat the oven to 350°F.

2. In a large bowl, cream the eggs, honey, oil, and applesauce until fluffy. Add the almond meal, cocoa powder, baking powder, walnuts, and zucchini and mix thoroughly.

3. Line a cake tin or loaf pan with parchment paper and pour in the mixture.

4. Bake in the oven for 50 to 60 minutes until a toothpick inserted in the middle comes out clean.

PER SERVING   Calories 240   Total carbohydrates 23.2g   Fat 16g
Protein 6.7g   Sodium 25mg   Sugar 19g

*See page 9 for quick ingredient substitutes and online retailer information

PUMPKIN CAKES

MAKES 6 SERVINGS   *Prep time: 15 minutes* • *Cook time: 25 minutes*

These muffins are a great combination of sweet treat and healthy snack. The pumpkin flavor and apple pie spice make it feel like autumn any time of the year.

1½ cups almond flour*

1 cup pumpkin purée

3 large eggs

1 teaspoon ground cinnamon

1 teaspoon apple pie spice

¼ teaspoon salt

½ teaspoon coconut oil

5 tablespoons honey

½ tablespoon almond butter

1. Preheat the oven to 350°F.

2. Line a muffin tin with paper liners. In a large mixing bowl, combine all of the ingredients and mix well. Pour the batter into the muffin tin.

3. Bake in the oven for 25 minutes.

PER SERVING Calories 243   Total carbohydrates 23.4g   Fat 15.4g
Protein 8.8g   Sodium 145mg   Sugar 16.3g

*See page 9 for quick ingredient substitutes and online retailer information

BERRY NUT COOKIES

MAKES 8 SERVINGS   *Prep time: 15 minutes • Cook time: 15 minutes*

Filled with chopped dates and cashew butter, these cookies are so rich, they will help fill you up quickly. The dried cranberries add a bit of tang—and a boost of antioxidants for good measure.

½ cup cashew butter

¼ cup dried cranberries

¼ cup chopped almonds

1 tablespoon coconut oil

1 egg

2 tablespoons pitted, chopped dates

1 tablespoon honey

1. Preheat the oven to 350°F.

2. In a medium mixing bowl, mix all of the ingredients together until thoroughly combined. Place spoonfuls of the dough onto a greased baking sheet.

3. Bake for about 12 minutes, until the cookies smell toasted. Allow to cool and harden before serving.

PER SERVING Calories 160   Total carbohydrates 12g   Fat 11.7g
Protein 4.3g   Sodium 11mg   Sugar 11g

COOKIE DOUGH SENSATION

MAKES 4 SERVINGS *Prep time: 10 minutes* • *Cook time: None*

Admit it: One of the best parts of making cookies is snacking on the dough long before it makes it to the baking sheet. Here is one way to indulge yourself and still stick to the basic paleo principles. (Some people believe chickpeas are paleo, some don't—so it's up to you.)

1 cup cooked chickpeas (garbanzos)

½ cup almond butter

2 tablespoons agave nectar*

1½ teaspoons vanilla extract

½ cup dark chocolate chips

1. In a blender, blend all ingredients except the chocolate chips.

2. Transfer the dough to a bowl. Fold the chocolate chips into the dough— and then, guess what? Eat by the spoonful!

PER SERVING Calories 396   Total carbohydrates 41.3g   Fat 23.2g
Protein 11.9g   Sodium 330mg   Sugar 34.3g

See page 9 for quick ingredient substitutes and online retailer information

DONUT DELIGHTS

MAKES 12 SERVINGS   *Prep time: 15 minutes • Cook time: 25 minutes*

And you thought donuts were on the no-no list! Try these and see how they do to help satisfy that sweet craving. The centers contain a surprise burst of raspberry jam. They're made in a muffin tin rather than being shaped like your average donut, but no one in your household will mind a bit.

½ cup applesauce

½ cup coconut oil, melted

3 eggs

3 tablespoons honey

1 tablespoon vanilla extract

½ cup coconut flour

½ teaspoon salt

¼ teaspoon baking soda

1 tablespoon almond milk

½ cup pure raspberry jam (low sugar)

1. Preheat the oven to 350°F. Line a dozen muffin cups with paper liners.

2. In a food processor, blend the applesauce, oil, eggs, honey, and vanilla. Transfer the mixture to a large mixing bowl and stir in the coconut flour, salt, and baking soda to form a solid batter. If it's too thick, add a little almond milk.

3. Fill the muffin cups about two-thirds full with batter, and then spoon jam into each cup. Bake for 25 minutes.

PER SERVING Calories 197   Total carbohydrates 21.7g   Fat 11.6g
Protein 3g   Sodium 142mg   Sugar 16.4g

CHOCOLATE ON TOP

MAKES 10 SERVINGS   *Prep time: 10 minutes* • *Cook time: None*

Have you ever made a batch of brownies, cookies, or cake and wished you had some frosting to add to the top? Here is a recipe for chocolate frosting that's paleo friendly—use it as you will (and certainly lick all the spoons when you're done!).

2 avocados, peeled and pitted
½ cup cocoa powder
½ cup honey
2 tablespoons coconut oil
1 teaspoon vanilla extract
½ teaspoon salt

1. In a food processor, blend all of the ingredients until smooth.

2. Frost away!

PER SERVING Calories 151   Total carbohydrates 19.8g   Fat 9.2g
Protein 1.7g   Sodium 121mg   Sugar 15.4g

A DELICIOUS MUG

MAKES 1 SERVING   *Prep time: 5 minutes • Cook time: 2 minutes*

This amazingly easy recipe is the perfect solution to that gnawing need for a quick bit of chocolate. If you want to make it extra flavorful, add a drop or two of coffee-flavored extract.

3 tablespoons dark chocolate chips
1 tablespoon olive oil
2 tablespoons coconut flour*
2 tablespoons water
⅛ teaspoon baking soda
1 egg

1. In a microwave-safe mug, combine the chocolate chips and oil. Heat in the microwave on high for 20 to 30 seconds until the chips are melted.

2. Stir in the coconut flour, water, and baking soda until combined. Add the egg and mix thoroughly.

3. Return the mug to the microwave and heat on high for 1½ minutes. Let it stand for 2 minutes before eating.

PER SERVING   Calories 467   Total carbohydrates 40.3g   Fat 30.9g
Protein 11.6g   Sodium 232mg   Sugar 26.2g

* See page 9 for quick ingredient substitutes and online retailer information

LUSCIOUS LEMON BARS

MAKES 4 SERVINGS   *Prep time: 10 minutes* • *Cook time: 20 minutes*

Lemon bars are the ideal blend of sweet and tart. This paleo-fied recipe makes them healthy, too.

For the bars:

1 cup almond meal*

3 tablespoons lemon juice

4 dates, pitted

For the filling:

6 tablespoons lemon juice

Zest of 1 lemon

1 tablespoon honey

2 eggs

To make the bars:

1. Preheat the oven to 350°F. Line muffin cups with paper liners.

2. In a food processor, blend the almond meal, 3 tablespoons lemon juice, and dates. Press the mixture firmly into the bottoms of the tins to form the crust.

3. Bake 10 to 12 minutes until lightly golden brown.

To make the filling:

1. In a saucepan over low heat, heat the 6 tablespoons lemon juice, zest, and honey. Simmer for 2 minutes. In a small bowl, beat the eggs and slowly add them to the simmering mix as you whisk briskly.

2. Remove from the heat and allow to cool for 5 minutes; then pour the filling into the shells. Chill in the refrigerator for at least 1 hour.

PER SERVING   Calories 244   Total carbohydrates 19.9g   Fat 16.6g
Protein 9.5g   Sodium 46mg   Sugar 15.4g

*See page 9 for quick ingredient substitutes and online retailer information

BANANA BREAD

MAKES 4 TO 5 SERVINGS   *Prep time: 15 minutes • Cook time: 45 minutes*

Dense, moist, sweetened bread can be the most delicious snack of all. Pair this one with a hot cup of coffee or tea.

Cooking spray

2 cups almond flour*

1 tablespoon ground cinnamon

1 teaspoon baking soda

2 eggs

½ cup water

1 teaspoon almond extract

¼ cup agave syrup*

2 ripe bananas, mashed

½ teaspoon vanilla bean paste
  (optional)*

1. Preheat the oven to 350°F.

2. Spray a loaf pan with cooking spray. In a large mixing bowl, combine the almond flour, cinnamon, and baking soda. In a medium mixing bowl, beat the eggs; then mix in the water, almond extract, agave syrup, mashed bananas, and vanilla bean paste.

3. Add the banana mixture to the flour mixture, and mix thoroughly. Pour the batter into the pan.

4. Bake for 45 minutes until crisp around the edges.

PER SERVING   Calories 244   Total carbohydrates 19.9g   Fat 16.6g
Protein 9.5g   Sodium 46mg   Sugar 15.4g

See page 9 for quick ingredient substitutes and online retailer information

GUILT-FREE COFFEE CAKE

MAKES 8 SERVINGS   *Prep time: 25 minutes • Cook time: 50 minutes*

A slice of coffee cake alongside a hot cup of coffee can be a wonderful solution to a snack attack. Here's a way to make a traditional baked goods and still be good. It takes a little extra effort, but it's definitely worth it.

For the topping:

Coconut oil

¾ cup chopped walnuts

3 tablespoons honey

1 teaspoon ground cinnamon

2 tablespoons coconut flour*

¼ cup cold unsalted butter,
   cut into cubes

For the fruit layer and crust:

2 pears, peeled and thinly sliced

1 apple, peeled and thinly sliced

2 teaspoon lemon juice

½ cup unsalted butter, softened

¼ cup honey

5 eggs

¾ cup coconut flour*

¾ cup coconut milk

¼ cup arrowroot powder*

1 teaspoon vanilla extract

¾ teaspoon baking powder

½ teaspoon baking soda

½ teaspoon salt

To make the topping:

1. Preheat the oven to 350°F.

2. Wrap the bottom of a springform pan in foil and grease the pan with oil.

3. In a medium bowl, stir together the walnuts, 3 tablespoons honey, and cinnamon. In another bowl, add 2 tablespoons coconut flour, and cut ¼ cup cold butter into the flour until it has the texture of coarse crumbs. Add the walnut mixture to the butter mixture and combine well. Set the topping aside.

---

* See page 9 for quick ingredient substitutes and online retailer information

To make the fruit layer and crust:

1. In a large bowl, mix the pears, apples, and lemon juice. In another bowl, beat ½ cup softened butter, ¼ cup honey, and the eggs together. Whisk the coconut flour, coconut milk, arrowroot powder, vanilla, baking powder, baking soda, and salt into the egg mixture until the batter is smooth.

2. Pour half of the batter into the pan. Spread the fruit in a layer over it, and then pour the remaining batter over the fruit. Top with the walnut mixture.

3. Bake for 50 to 55 minutes until done. Cool for 1 hour before serving.

PER SERVING Calories 528   Total carbohydrates 48.2g   Fat 35.4g
Protein 10g   Sodium 285mg   Sugar 34.6g

COCONUT COBBLER

MAKES 4 SERVINGS   *Prep time: 5 minutes* • *Cook time: 5 minutes*

Traditional fruit cobbler has lots of sugar and usually contains oatmeal. This paleo version is amazingly simple and fast, yet still so tasty! For best results, make it in the summer when the berries are at their peak.

2 cups mixed fresh berries
1 teaspoon water
½ cup coconut milk
1 tablespoon ground cinnamon
½ cup almond meal*

1. In a pan over medium heat, cook the berries, covered, for 5 minutes until they soften (if they look at all dry, add a teaspoon of water). Remove from the heat.

2. In a mixing bowl, whisk the coconut milk and cinnamon together.

3. Place the berries in a bowl, pour the milk over them, and sprinkle the almond meal on top.

PER SERVING   Calories 142   Total carbohydrates 12.2g   Fat 8.9g
Protein 6.7g   Sodium 6mg   Sugar 7.8g

* See page 9 for quick ingredient substitutes and online retailer information

DIY CHOCOLATE

MAKES 8 SERVINGS   *Prep time: 10 minutes • Cook time: None*

Chocolate is good in any form—including just as chocolate! Make your own and eat it as is, or use it however you like. Plan to do a lot of licking of spoons and bowls.

½ cup coconut oil
½ cup cocoa powder
3 tablespoons honey
½ teaspoon vanilla extract

1. In a saucepan over low to medium heat, melt the oil. Stir in the cocoa powder, honey, and vanilla until well mixed.

2. Pour the mixture into a candy mold and refrigerate for 1 hour until chilled.

PER SERVING Calories 157   Total carbohydrates 9.4g   Fat 14.7g
Protein 1.1g   Sodium 1mg   Sugar 6.8g

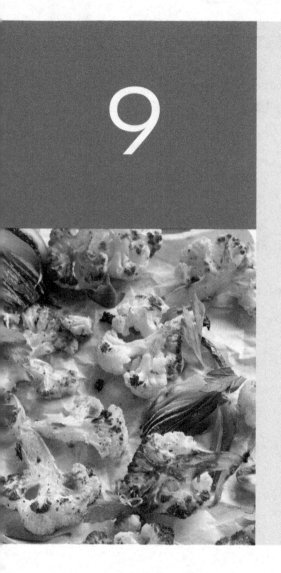

9

KEEPIN' IT LIGHT

Perhaps one of the best things about the paleo diet is that it doesn't focus on calories nearly as much as other diets. Most paleo eaters never give calories much thought at all. (Can you picture a caveman keeping track of how much he has eaten and cutting back if he hits a certain number?) However, if you're focusing more on the weight-loss aspect of the lifestyle rather than just overall health, these snack recipes can be helpful. They are high in nutrients, but low in calories.

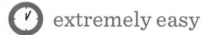

CUCUMBER CUPS

MAKES 16 SERVINGS   *Prep time: 15 minutes • Cook time: None*

These low-calorie cucumber cups are fresh and easy to put together for a quick snack. How can you improve on that? The ham provides protein, and the curry powder gives it a little kick. Perfect for a mid-afternoon work break or an after-school snack.

16 half-inch-thick slices of cucumber
½ cup coarsely chopped cooked ham
3 tablespoons mayonnaise
2 teaspoons Dijon mustard
½ teaspoon curry powder

1. Using a melon baller (or an ice cream scoop), scoop out the center of each cucumber slice. This leaves the bottom intact, forming a small cup.

2. Place the ham, mayonnaise, mustard, and curry powder in a food processor, and pulse until minced and thoroughly mixed.

3. Spoon about 2 teaspoons of filling into each cucumber cup and serve.

PER SERVING   Calories 23   Total carbohydrates 1.1g   Fat 1.7g
Protein 0.9g   Sodium 89mg   Sugar 0g

CHICKEN KABOBS

MAKES 12 SERVINGS   *Prep time: 15 minutes • Cook time: 15 minutes*

This recipe works best on a grill, so make it on a summer afternoon as an appetizer, or as a snack for a pack of party guests. The original recipe calls for soy sauce, which many paleo dieters avoid, so it's replaced here with coconut aminos. You'll need skewers to make these kabobs.

¼ cup olive oil

⅓ cup honey

⅓ cup coconut aminos*

¼ teaspoon black pepper

8 boneless, skinless chicken breast halves, cut into 1-inch cubes

2 garlic cloves

5 small onions, cut into 2-inch pieces

2 red peppers, cut into 2-inch pieces

1. In a large mixing bowl, whisk together the oil, honey, coconut aminos, and black pepper. Take out a little of this marinade to use for basting the kabobs while they cook. Add the chicken, garlic, onions, and peppers to the bowl, and marinate for at least 2 hours in the refrigerator.

2. Preheat the grill to high heat. Drain the marinade from the bowl and discard.

3. Carefully thread the chicken and vegetables alternately onto the skewers. Place the skewers on the lightly oiled grill grate. Grill for 12 to 15 minutes, turning and brushing frequently with the reserved marinade.

PER SERVING   Calories 178   Total carbohydrates 12.4g   Fat 6.6g
Protein 17.4g   Sodium 145mg   Sugar 5.1g

See page 9 for quick ingredient substitutes and online retailer information

LOW-CARB EGGCAKES

MAKES 18 TO 20 SERVINGS   *Prep time: 20 minutes* • *Cook time: 25 minutes*

These savory "cupcakes" have a great combination of flavors—eggs, bacon, roasted peppers, and more. Try them for breakfast or an afternoon snack that will hit the spot. Take a few to work and simply pop them in the microwave to reheat.

12 eggs
1 green onion
2 zucchini
8 slices bacon
½ jar roasted red and yellow peppers
2 cups spinach
Salt and pepper

1. Preheat oven to 350°F. Grease two muffin pans.

2. In a large mixing bowl, whisk the eggs well. Place the onion, zucchini, bacon, and peppers in a food processor, and process until chopped. Add the mixture to the eggs. Process the spinach until finely chopped, and then add to the egg mixture. Season with salt and pepper and mix thoroughly.

3. Fill the muffin pans with the mixture. Bake for 20 to 25 minutes, until the eggs are set.

PER SERVING Calories 60   Total carbohydrates 1.1g   Fat 3.9g
Protein 4.8g   Sodium 105.4mg   Sugar 0.6g

POPCORN CAULIFLOWER

MAKES 4 SERVINGS   *Prep time: 10 minutes* • *Cook time: 60 minutes*

Most of the time when cauliflower is served, it is steamed—and often for far too long. This recipe roasts it, which gives this underestimated vegetable a unique and wonderful flavor.

1 head cauliflower

4 tablespoons olive oil

1 teaspoon salt

1. Preheat the oven to 425°F.

2. Cut the head of cauliflower into florets about the size of golf balls. Discard the core and leaves. In a small bowl, whisk together the oil and salt and then pour it over the florets.

3. Line a baking sheet with parchment paper and spread the pieces across it. Roast in the oven for 1 hour, turning the pieces three to four times, until they are all golden brown. Keep in mind that the browner the pieces get, the sweeter and more intense the flavor will be.

PER SERVING   Calories 155   Total carbohydrates 7.5g   Fat 14.5g
Protein 3g   Sodium 625mg   Sugar 0g

PALEO JAMBALAYA

MAKES 6 SERVINGS   *Prep time: 15 minutes* • *Cook time: 30 minutes*

A traditional favorite in many cultures, jambalaya can often be packed with carbohydrates. This version keeps the flavor, but loses the carbs. Make it for a meal, and then have it for a snack for the next week.

1 tablespoon olive oil

1 tablespoon butter

1 large onion, chopped

2 andouille sausages, halved
   lengthwise and cut in ¼-inch
   half moons

6 garlic cloves, finely chopped

One 14-ounce can crushed tomatoes

3 green bell peppers, seeded and diced

2 zucchini, diced

2 tablespoons Cajun seasoning

1 teaspoon hot sauce

1 cup chicken broth

1 pound chicken breast, cooked, cooled,
   and chopped

1 pound shrimp, peeled, deveined, and
   cooked

1. In a large saucepan over medium heat, heat the oil and butter. Add the onion and sausage and stir for about 10 minutes, until the onion browns. Add the garlic and cook another 1 to 2 minutes. Mix in the tomatoes, peppers, zucchini, seasoning, hot sauce, and broth.

2. Bring the mixture to a boil, and then reduce to a simmer. Cook uncovered for about 15 minutes, until the mixture is thickened.

3. Add the meat and simmer another 1 to 2 minutes, until heated through.

PER SERVING   Calories 260   Total carbohydrates 14.5g   Fat 8.5g
Protein 31.8g   Sodium 974mg   Sugar 0g

SMOKY SOUP

MAKES 6 SERVINGS   *Prep time: 25 minutes • Cook time: 2 minutes*

Soup as a snack? Absolutely! It's hot. It's filling. It's fast. It's delicious. What else do you need? The paprika is what brings out the flavors, so make sure you have some in the spice cabinet before making this recipe.

1 medium head cauliflower

1 small onion, finely chopped

1 tablespoon olive oil

3 cups chicken broth

1 to 2 teaspoons smoked paprika

Salt and pepper

2 slices cooked bacon, crumbled

¼ cup chopped parsley

1. In a pot of water on high heat, steam the cauliflower on a steaming tray until tender. Meanwhile, in a skillet over medium-high heat, sauté the onion in the oil until translucent.

2. When the cauliflower is done, purée half of it in a blender, along with the onion, broth, and paprika. Season with salt and pepper. Add the remaining cauliflower, plus the bacon and parsley, and blend again for 1 minute.

3. Pour the soup into a large serving bowl. If it's not hot enough to serve, put in the microwave on high for 1 minute.

PER SERVING   Calories 64   Total carbohydrates 6.9g   Fat 3.3g
Protein 2.6g   Sodium 491mg   Sugar 3.3g

DR. SEUSS EGGS

MAKES 12 SERVINGS · *Prep time: 30 minutes* · *Cook time: 10 minutes*

Make these right before you're going to serve them because avocados tend to look a little funky after being exposed to the air for a while. Green eggs are okay; discolored brown ones, not so much.

6 eggs, hard-boiled

½ avocado

¼ cup mayonnaise

1 teaspoon brown mustard

½ teaspoon celery salt

1 scallion, minced

2 dashes hot sauce

Paprika

1. In a pot on the stove, hard-boil the eggs in water. When done, slice them in half and scoop the yolks into a mixing bowl. Set the whites aside.

2. With a fork, lightly mash the yolks. Scoop the avocado out of its shell and add it to the yolks. Transfer the mixture to a food processor, add the rest of the ingredients, and process until very creamy and smooth.

3. Stuff the mixture into the egg white halves and sprinkle with paprika. It's green eggs today!

PER SERVING Calories 86 Total carbohydrates 1g Fat 8g
Protein 3g Sodium 580mg Sugar 0g

PINEAPPLE PIZZAZZ

MAKES 4 SERVINGS   *Prep time: 5 minutes* • *Cook time: None*

You will never look at pineapple the same way again after this unusual twist on flavors. Recipes don't get much simpler than this!

2 cups fresh pineapple chunks
¼ cup coconut aminos*
Red pepper flakes

1. Place the pineapple chunks on a plate, and put a toothpick in each one.

2. Put a bowl of the coconut aminos and pepper flakes next to them for dipping.

PER SERVING Calories 38   Total carbohydrates 10g   Fat 0g
Protein 0g   Sodium 15mg   Sugar 8g

*See page 9 for quick ingredient substitutes and online retailer information

CINFLOWER BALLS

When you combine seeds, raisins, and cinnamon, the result tastes great without a lot of calories. Sunflower seeds provide a variety of nutritional benefits, too, including significant amounts of vitamin E, magnesium, and selenium.

1 cup sunflower seeds

¼ cup raisins

¼ teaspoon ground cinnamon

2 tablespoons coconut oil, melted

1 tablespoon water

1. In a food processor, blend the seeds, raisins, and cinnamon until finely ground. Add the oil and water and process until it forms a stiff dough.

2. Form into 18 balls about the size of Ping-Pong balls. Eat right away or store in the refrigerator for later.

PER SERVING Calories 65   Total carbohydrates 3g   Fat 5g
Protein 2g   Sodium 1mg   Sugar 2.7g

ZIPPY DIP

MAKES 12 SERVINGS   *Prep time: 10 minutes* • *Cook time: None*

This is a dip that's high in flavor (hence the zippy!) as well as fiber, calcium, and iron. Meanwhile, it's low in calories, fat, and carbs. Try it on paleo crackers or with some crunchy veggies.

1 cup pitted green olives
Two 15-ounce jars of artichoke hearts, drained
1 tablespoon capers, drained
1 garlic clove
1 tablespoon fresh parsley
¼ teaspoon red pepper flakes
Salt
Olive oil (optional)

1. In a food processor, mix the first six ingredients until combined, yet still chunky. Season with salt to taste.

2. To add extra flavor, feel free to add ¼ cup of olive oil as well.

PER SERVING   Calories 46   Total carbohydrates 5g   Fat 3g
Protein 2g   Sodium 424mg   Sugar 0g

ROE AND ROUNDS

MAKES 20 SERVINGS   *Prep time: 10 minutes* • *Cook time: None*

Need a fancy snack to serve to friends and family? This one requires a couple of exotic ingredients, so pull it out when you want to make an impression on seafood fans.

2 cucumbers, sliced into rounds

1 sheet nori, cut into small squares*

1 avocado, cut into small chunks

2 ounces pink salmon roe*

1. Line up the cucumber rounds on a serving platter.

2. Put a square of nori on top of each round. Top with a chunk of avocado and a little dab of salmon roe.

PER SERVING Calories 120   Total carbohydrates 8g   Fat 9g
Protein 6g   Sodium 2.3mg   Sugar 0g

*See page 9 for quick ingredient substitutes and online retailer information

BLOODY MARY 'MATOES

MAKES 16 SERVINGS   *Prep time: 3 minutes • Cook time: None (overnight soaking)*

This recipe is excellent for a cocktail party or a get-together for a big game or the holidays. In other words, great for adults, but not for kids. Note how long the soaking period is so you can be prepared.

1 pint cherry tomatoes
1 cup pepper-flavored vodka
2 tablespoons hot pepper sauce
2 tablespoons lemon pepper
2 tablespoons celery salt

1. After removing any stems from the tomatoes, place them in a shallow bowl, and pour the vodka over them until completely covered. Stir in the hot pepper sauce and then cover the bowl. Chill in the refrigerator overnight.

2. When it's time to serve, mix the lemon pepper and celery salt in a dish and set aside. Serve the tomatoes floating in the vodka. Put toothpicks out so people can spear the tomatoes and then roll them in the seasoning before munching.

PER SERVING Calories 40   Total carbohydrates 1.1g   Fat 0.2g
Protein 0.2g   Sodium 742mg   Sugar 0g

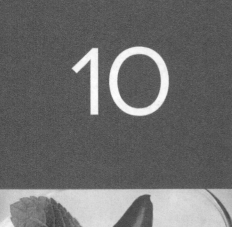

10

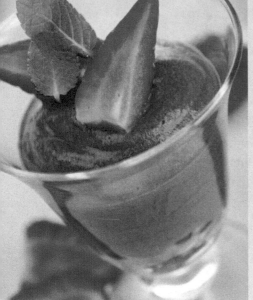

TIME FOR DESSERT

The wonderful thing about dessert is that even if you're so full you've loosened your belt and you're squirming to get more comfortable in your chair, somehow there is still enough room for it! Dessert is a sweet and delicious luxury, so we tend to enjoy every single crumb. Here's a great variety of temptations to try after dinner, at midnight, or—why not? even for breakfast!

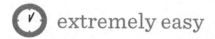

MAPLE STRAWBERRIES

MAKES 4 SERVINGS   *Prep time: 5 minutes* • *Cook time: None*

This is incredibly fast and simple, and best made in the summer when strawberries are bursting with flavor. They are divine when combined with maple.

1 pound fresh strawberries
3 teaspoons maple syrup

1. Wash the berries and put them in a serving bowl.

2. Fill a custard cup with the syrup and serve it alongside the berries. Have people dip their berries in the syrup.

PER SERVING Calories 66   Total carbohydrates 16g   Fat 0g
Protein 1g   Sodium 0mg   Sugar 9g

TROPICAL
ICE CREAM

MAKES 6 SERVINGS   *Prep time: 15 minutes* • *Cook time: None*

Dairy-free ice cream may sound difficult to make, but this recipe proves how easily it can be done. The pineapple and coconut give it tropical flair.

4 cups frozen banana slices
1 cup frozen pineapple chunks
One 14-ounce can coconut milk
Juice of 1 lime
Pinch of salt

1. Thaw the banana and pineapple at room temperature for about 5 minutes.

2. In a food processor, blend the banana, pineapple, and coconut milk for 1 minute, until smooth. Add the lime juice and the salt and process again.

3. Line a baking dish with plastic wrap and pour the mixture in it. Freeze until it is the consistency of ice cream, 40 to 45 minutes.

PER SERVING Calories 246   Total carbohydrates 32.4g   Fat 14.3g
Protein 2.7g   Sodium 77mg   Sugar 16g

BANANA CHOCOLATE CHIP COOKIES

MAKES 16 SERVINGS   *Prep time: 10 minutes • Cook time: 15 minutes*

Missing those Tollhouse treats? Try these cookies instead. They're much healthier for you and totally delicious.

½ cup coconut flour*
½ teaspoon baking soda
8 tablespoons coconut oil
1 very ripe banana
2 large eggs
1½ teaspoons vanilla extract
¾ cup dark chocolate chips

1. Preheat the oven to 350°F.

2. In a large mixing bowl, combine the coconut flour and baking soda. In another bowl, mix the oil, banana, eggs, and vanilla. Stir the wet mixture into the dry mixture and combine well; then stir in the chocolate chips. Place the batter by the teaspoonful on a greased baking sheet.

3. Bake for 12 minutes until the edges are golden brown.

PER SERVING Calories 113   Total carbohydrates 6.8g   Fat 9.7g
Protein 1.2g   Sodium 49.1mg   Sugar 5.2g

*See page 9 for quick ingredient substitutes and online retailer information

PECAN PRIZE ICE CREAM

MAKES 2 SERVINGS *Prep time: 5 minutes • Cook time: None*

There can never be enough recipes for ice cream. Here's one that includes the wonderful addition of pecans, and uses smooth, creamy banana for the base.

2 bananas, cut up and frozen
1 tablespoon agave syrup* (optional)
1 teaspoon vanilla
Pinch of salt
½ cup pecans

1. Thaw the bananas at room temperature for about 10 minutes.

2. Place the bananas, syrup (if using), vanilla, and salt in a food processor, and process until smooth. Add the pecans and pulse a few times to coarsely chop them. Serve immediately.

PER SERVING   Calories 300   Total carbohydrates 30.9g   Fat 20g
Protein 3.7g   Sodium 292mg   Sugar 15.7g

* See page 9 for quick ingredient substitutes and online retailer information

PERSIMMON PIE

MAKES 8 SERVINGS   *Prep time: 30 minutes* • *Cook time: None*

Persimmons are one of those fruits that most people avoid in the produce section because they have no idea how to tell when one is ripe and how to eat it. One bite of an unripe persimmon is enough to turn you off forever (can you say pucker?), so make sure yours are ripe. They will look like they're about to split, fall apart, and be thrown away.

½ teaspoon olive oil

3 cups pecans

20 pitted dates

¼ cup agave nectar*

6 very ripe persimmons

2 tablespoons chopped pecans, plus more for garnish

1 teaspoon cinnamon for garnish

1. Lightly grease a pie pan with the oil.

2. In a food processor, blend the pecans and dates for 1 minute, until finely ground. Add the agave and blend for 30 seconds. Press this mixture evenly into the pie pan.

3. Peel and pit the persimmons; then purée them in the food processor until smooth. Pour over the crust and flatten evenly. Garnish with pecans and cinnamon.

PER SERVING Calories 411   Total carbohydrates 36g   Fat 31.2g
Protein 4.6g   Sodium 0.5mg   Sugar 28.3g

*See page 9 for quick ingredient substitutes and online retailer information

PINEAPPLE ON THE GRILL

MAKES 4 SERVINGS   *Prep time: 10 minutes • Cook time: 10 minutes*

Cooking on the grill always seems to give food a fabulous flavor, and that is certainly true for this dessert. While this grilled pineapple is great served on the side of a juicy steak, it's also fantastic by itself as a snack.

2 tablespoons honey

2 tablespoons dark rum

½ teaspoon ground cinnamon

4 teaspoons coconut oil

12 ounces fresh pineapple, in chunks

1. In a small mixing bowl, combine the honey, rum, and cinnamon.

2. Tear four 12-inch squares of aluminum foil and slightly turn each one up on the edges. Place 1 teaspoon of the oil in each one. Divide the pineapple chunks evenly among the foil pieces and drizzle them with the honey-rum mixture. Fold the foil so the edges come together, and then roll up the ends.

3. Put them on the grill for 10 minutes, turning over about halfway through. Let them cool and serve warm.

PER SERVING Calories 87   Total carbohydrates 9g   Fat 5g
Protein 0g   Sodium 0mg   Sugar 14.5g

IN A GLAZE

MAKES 6 SERVINGS   *Prep time: 30 minutes* • *Cook time: 10 minutes*

This is a fun dessert, but watch it carefully on the stove top—the line between toasted and burned is very, very thin. Walnuts have never tasted so good!

1½ cups walnuts
Boiling water
1 tablespoon honey
½ teaspoon vanilla
Coconut oil

1. Place the walnuts in a heatproof bowl and cover them with boiling water; let stand for 4 or 5 minutes. Drain well, and then add the honey and toss well. Add the vanilla and toss again.

2. Spread the walnuts on a plate and allow to dry for 1 to 2 hours.

3. Using a heavy skillet, heat the oil over medium heat, and fry the walnuts a handful at a time until they are crisp. Don't walk away—they burn easily. Cool and store—or gobble them all up right away.

PER SERVING Calories 201   Total carbohydrates 7g   Fat 18g
Protein 8g   Sodium 0g   Sugar 2.9g

NUTTY CEREAL

Prep time: 10 minutes • Cook time: 30 to 40 minutes

You can eat this with paleo yogurt, cover it in coconut milk, float it in almond milk—or just munch on it by the handful. This is pretty rich and high in carbohydrates, calories, and fat grams, so enjoy, but eat in moderation.

½ cup pumpkin purée

½ cup coconut oil

⅓ cup honey

1 teaspoon vanilla

2 tablespoons ground cinnamon

1 tablespoon ground nutmeg

⅛ teaspoon ground cloves

⅛ teaspoon ground ginger

½ cup sliced almonds

½ cup pecans, chopped

½ cup pumpkin seeds

8 dates, chopped

⅓ cup shredded unsweetened coconut

1. Preheat the oven to 325°F. Line a baking sheet with parchment paper.

2. In a large bowl, mix the pumpkin purée, oil, honey, vanilla, and spices together. Add the nuts, seeds, dates, and coconut, and mix well. Spread evenly on the lined baking sheet.

3. Bake for 30 to 40 minutes, taking it out halfway through to mix. Allow it to cool before serving, which also allows it to get crunchy.

PER SERVING Calories 676   Total carbohydrates 48.8g   Fat 54.1g
Protein 9.6g   Sodium 24mg   Sugar 37.6g

CHOCOLATE PUDDING INDULGENCE

MAKES 4 SERVINGS · *Prep time: 20 minutes* · *Cook time: None*

What does an avocado have to do with chocolate pudding? More than you might think. Avocados help recipes turn out thicker, smoother, and creamier, and that is certainly the case with this one.

2 ripe avocados

1 cup cocoa powder

½ cup honey

¼ teaspoon French vanilla liquid stevia*

8 strawberries, diced

1. Cut the avocados in half, remove the pits, and scoop out the flesh. Put it in the food processor, and add the cocoa powder, honey, and stevia. Process until it is as smooth and thick as pudding.

2. Spoon the pudding into dessert bowls and garnish with the strawberries.

PER SERVING Calories 676   Total carbohydrates 48.8g   Fat 54.1g
Protein 9.6g   Sodium 24mg   Sugar 37.6g

* *See page 9 for quick ingredient substitutes and online retailer information*

ROASTED PEARS

MAKES 4 SERVINGS   *Prep time: 20 minutes • Cook time: 1 hour*

While some of the recipes in the book were designed to be made during the summer, this one is geared for autumn. If you've never tasted roasted pears before, you're in for a treat!

2 ripe pears
1 tablespoon maple syrup
½ teaspoon ground cinnamon
¼ cup chopped walnuts

1. Preheat the oven to 350°F. Grease a baking dish.

2. Cut the pears in half, scoop out the cores, and remove the stems. Put the pears in the baking dish, cut side up. Put ½ tablespoon maple syrup in the hollow of each pear half and spread some over the cut surfaces as well. Sprinkle each half with the cinnamon.

3. Bake for 1 hour. During the last 10 minutes, spread the walnuts in an ovenproof pan and roast them alongside the pears.

4. Remove the pears and walnuts from the oven at the same time. Sprinkle the walnuts on the top of the pears and serve.

PER SERVING Calories 123   Total carbohydrates 20g   Fat 5g
Protein 2g   Sodium 0mg   Sugar 0.5g

PALEO GINGERBREAD

MAKES 16 SERVINGS *Prep time: 20 minutes* • *Cook time: 30 to 35 minutes*

The flavor of gingerbread is one that some people absolutely love. If you're a fan, check out this recipe, even if it's not the holiday season. Go ahead, it's okay—it's totally paleo!

1 cup almond meal*

¼ cup flaxseed meal*

¼ cup coconut meal*

¼ teaspoon salt

1 teaspoon baking soda

2 teaspoons ground ginger

1 teaspoon ground cinnamon

¼ cup coconut oil, melted

¼ cup honey

32 drops liquid stevia*

½ cup coconut milk or plain yogurt

2 eggs

1. Preheat the oven to 350°F. Grease a baking pan.

2. In a mixing bowl, combine the dry ingredients until thoroughly mixed. In another mixing bowl, mix together the oil, honey, stevia, and milk. Crack the eggs into the wet ingredients and mix well. Pour this mixture into the dry ingredients and whisk thoroughly.

3. Pour the batter into the pan and bake for 30 to 35 minutes.

PER SERVING Calories 123 Total carbohydrates 11g Fat 7g
Protein 6g Sodium 10mg Sugar 5g

See page 9 for quick ingredient substitutes and online retailer information

BAKED CUSTARD

MAKES 6 SERVINGS   *Prep time: 5 minutes • Cook time: 4 hours*

This is so good you can eat it for breakfast, dessert, or a snack. It requires a slow cooker and has to chill overnight.

14 fluid ounces unsweetened coconut milk
3 tablespoons honey
¼ teaspoon French vanilla liquid stevia*
5 eggs
¼ teaspoon salt

1. Place all ingredients in a blender, and process until smooth. Pour the batter into a 1-quart Pyrex casserole dish.

2. Cover the dish with aluminum foil and place in a slow cooker. Fill the space around the dish with water, up to an inch from the rim. Cover the pot, set it on low, and cook for 4 hours.

3. Turn off the slow cooker, remove the lid, and let the water cool before you remove the casserole dish. Chill the dish overnight before serving.

PER SERVING   Calories 216   Total carbohydrates 11g   Fat 17g
Protein 6g   Sodium 48.4mg   Sugar 8.6g

*See page 9 for quick ingredient substitutes and online retailer information

SWEET AND DARK

MAKES 24 SERVINGS   *Prep time: 20 minutes • Cook time: 10 minutes*

With all of the savory and spice in many of the dishes in this book, you're going to need some sweetness for balance. Try this recipe—even people who aren't big fans of the paleo diet will fall for these cookies.

2 cups almond flour*

1/3 cup coconut flour*

2/3 cup shredded unsweetened coconut

1 egg

1/2 cup almond butter, softened

1/4 cup honey

1 1/2 teaspoons coconut oil, melted

1 teaspoon vanilla extract

3/4 cup dark chocolate chips

1. Preheat the oven to 350°F.

2. In a large mixing bowl, combine the flours and shredded coconut. In another bowl, beat the egg and slowly add the almond butter, honey, oil, and vanilla.

3. Once thoroughly mixed, add the wet mixture to the dry ingredients and mix until the dough is smooth. Add the chocolate chips and stir until just combined.

4. Put teaspoon-size balls of dough 1 inch apart on ungreased baking sheets and bake for about 10 minutes.

PER SERVING Calories 167   Total carbohydrates 12.7g   Fat 12.2g
Protein 4.2g   Sodium 29mg   Sugar 9.6g

See page 9 for quick ingredient substitutes and online retailer information

RECIPE INDEX

INDEX

A

agave nectar/syrup, 53, 122, 127, 151–152

almond butter, 16, 42, 45, 59, 88, 120, 122, 160

almond flour, 50, 53–55, 60–61, 69, 78–79, 114, 127, 160

almond meal, 20, 61, 85, 119, 126, 130, 158

almond milk, 13, 15, 20, 24–25, 67, 89, 123

almonds, 13, 43–44, 49, 53, 70, 88–89, 95

apple juice, 18, 55

apples/applesauce, 21, 55, 88, 119, 123, 128–129

apricots, dried, 55

artichoke hearts, 143

arugula, 92

avocados, 22, 24, 81, 90, 115, 124, 140, 144, 156

B

baby carrots, 28

bacon, 65, 83, 91–92, 95, 107, 109, 112, 115, 139

bananas, 12, 14, 17, 19, 21, 24, 59, 60, 67, 68, 127, 149–151

barbecue sauce, 84

bars, 40–55

beef, 76, 80, 103, 106, 108

bell peppers, 28, 80, 136

black raspberries, 14

blood sugar stabilization, 6

blue cheese, 83

blueberries, 14, 23, 46

broccoli florets, 28

Brussels sprouts, 64

buckwheat, dried, 55

burritos, 90

butternut squash, 31, 63

C

cakes, 120, 128–129

caraway seeds, 76

carrots, 28, 60, 106, 108, 113

cashew butter, 88, 121

cashews, 44

cauliflower, 28, 137, 139

celery stalks, 21, 28, 65, 93, 108

Cheddar cheese, 75

cherries, dried, 49

chicken, 110, 112–115, 135, 138

chicken breasts, 83, 113, 114, 115, 135, 138

chickpeas, 122

chili, 80

chips and dips, 26–39, 143

chocolate chips, dark, 122, 125, 150, 160

cocoa powder, unsweetened, 16, 45, 48–49, 68, 80, 105, 119, 124, 131, 156

coconut, 25, 44, 113

coconut aminos, 141

coconut flour, 50, 55, 125, 128–129, 150, 160

coconut milk, 12–14, 16, 51–52, 58, 63, 67, 89, 94, 96–98, 114, 128–130, 149, 159

coconut, unsweetened, 15, 46, 51–53, 55, 58, 155, 160

coconut water, 23

cookies, 70, 121, 150

cost factors, 7

CPSIA information can be obtained at www.ICGtesting.com
Printed in the USA
LVOW05*0152081015

457321LV00005BA/22/P

9 781623 155063